Unsafe at Any Dose:
The Chemical Contamination
of
Modern Medicine

Kevin B DiBacco

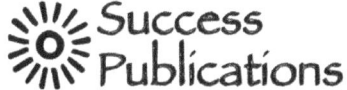

TABLE OF CONTENTS

Introduction: The Trust Trap 7
Chapter 1: Beyond the Active Ingredient 18
Chapter 2: The Manufacturing Web 33
Chapter 3: Regulatory Blind Spots 48
Chapter 4: The Inactive Ingredient Myth 68
Chapter 5: Colors, Flavors, and Preservatives 90
Chapter 6: Manufacturing Contaminants 109
Chapter 7: Generic vs. Brand Name Reality 130
Chapter 8: The Inspection Game 146
Chapter 9: Recalls You Never Heard About 168
Chapter 10: Over-the-Counter Dangers 183
Chapter 11: The Money Trail 200
Chapter 12: Reading Between the Lines 218
Chapter 13: Minimizing Your Risk 237
Chapter 14: The Path Forward 259
Conclusion: Your Journey Toward Pharmaceutical Safety . 277
Sources and Further Reading 283

Copyright © 2025 Kevin B. DiBacco
All rights reserved.

No part of this book may be reproduced, stored in a retrieval system, or transmitted in any form or by any means—electronic, mechanical, photocopying, recording, or otherwise—without the prior written permission of the copyright holder, except for brief quotations used in reviews, academic studies, or articles.

Disclaimer

The information presented in this book is intended for educational and informational purposes only. It reflects the author's research, investigative findings, and personal opinions at the time of writing. This book is not intended to provide medical advice or to be a substitute for consultation with a licensed medical professional.

Always seek the advice of a physician, pharmacist, or other qualified health provider with any questions you may have regarding medications, health conditions, or treatment plans. Never disregard professional medical advice or delay seeking treatment based on the content of this book.

While every effort has been made to verify the information provided, the author and publisher make no representations or warranties regarding the accuracy, applicability, or completeness of the content. They disclaim any liability or responsibility for any loss, injury, or damage that may occur as a result of following or applying any of the information presented herein.

References to real individuals, corporations, agencies, or products are for context only and do not imply endorsement or criticism unless expressly stated.

ABOUT THE AUTHOR

Kevin B. DiBacco is a bestselling author, award-winning filmmaker, and former USAF Security Forces veteran whose debut novel *Badge of Horror* is now being sold worldwide. With multiple international bestsellers to his name and seven traditional publishing deals secured, Kevin has established himself as a formidable voice across both fiction and nonfiction genres.

Over his 37-year career in filmmaking, Kevin's work was showcased at top-tier festivals including Sundance and Cannes, with international distribution in five major territories. But his most compelling story is his own: surviving a life-threatening brain surgery, undergoing a three-year recovery, and losing 60 pounds at age 62. Kevin's journey is a testament to unbreakable willpower, chronicled in his writings that inspire, educate, and empower.

His internationally recognized bestsellers include *Being Weird: Unleash Your Inner Weirdo and Conquer the World*(Viking House), *Single Band Workout* (Global Publishing Agency), and *The Lost Art of Logical Thinking* (Chelsea House Press). Kevin has secured publishing deals with prestigious houses including Viking House, Global Publishing Agency, Chelsea House Press, New Castle Publishing, Urban Viking Publishing UK, Staten House, Success Publications, and Tribune Publishing Company.

His acclaimed titles span diverse subjects:

- *Microplastics: Poisoning the People* – Global Publishing Agency
- *Bad Air: What Are We Breathing?* – Chelsea House Press
- *Fitness Decoded: Unlocking the Secrets to Healthiness & Happiness at Any Age!* – New Castle Publishing
- *Indie Filmmaking in the Real World* – Urban Viking Publishing UK

- *HYSOMETRICS* – Urban Viking Publishing UK
- *Hold the Power* – Urban Viking Publishing UK
- *Chemicals in Our Food* – Staten House
- *The Handshake: Around the World* – Success Publications
- *Powerlifting with Bands* – Urban Viking Publishing UK
- *Recharge: The Powernap* – Tribune Publishing Company

In nonfiction, Kevin has become known for delivering raw, practical, and inspiring content across genres ranging from fitness and mental health to environmental advocacy and media literacy. His powerful book *Depression: Understanding and Overcoming* reflects his personal battle with clinical depression, while his ISO QUICK STRENGTH program merges mental and physical resilience into one transformative system.

Now turning the page to fiction, *Badge of Horror* marks the start of a bold new chapter. Combining suspense, realism, and sharp insight, the novel is just the beginning of a storytelling legacy that bridges personal truth with compelling narrative.

Kevin's motto *"If you can see it, you can do it"* continues to fuel his work and inspire audiences around the world.

Introduction: The Trust Trap
A Patient's Awakening

I've been cut open more times than I care to count.

Eighteen surgeries, to be exact. Torn ACLs, shattered bones, damaged cartilage, reconstructed joints—the inevitable price of a lifetime spent pushing my body to its athletic limits. Each time I found myself in a hospital bed, a different doctor would appear with the same routine: explaining the procedure, discussing recovery time, and handing me a prescription for pain medication.

"Take two of every four hours," they'd say, barely glancing up from their prescription pad. "This will help with the pain."

But I started asking questions that apparently no one else was asking: "What exactly is in these pills? Where are they made? What are the side effects of taking them for weeks or months at a time?"

The answers I got were disturbing in their vagueness.

"It's just a standard pain reliever," one orthopedic surgeon told me after my fourteenth surgery. When I pressed for specifics about the inactive ingredients, he admitted he didn't actually know what else was in the medication he was prescribing. "The FDA approves them," he said with a shrug. "That's good enough for me."

But it wasn't good enough for me anymore.

The Prescription Treadmill

Over the years, I've been prescribed nearly every pain medication in existence: OxyContin, Percocet, Vicodin, Tramadol, Fentanyl patches, Morphine, Codeine, and dozens of others whose names I can barely pronounce. Each surgeon seemed to have their favorite, their go-to drug that they prescribed to every patient regardless of individual circumstances.

What struck me wasn't just the casual way these powerful substances were handed out—it was the complete absence of curiosity about what else these medications contained. The doctors focused entirely on the active ingredient, the part that would dull my pain, while completely ignoring the other 60-80% of each pill's contents.

After my twentieth surgery, I started declining the prescriptions. The pain was manageable, and something about swallowing chemical cocktails that no one could fully explain didn't sit right with me. My doctors thought I was crazy. "Why would you choose to be in pain?" they asked.

Because I was starting to suspect that the pain might be preferable to the unknown consequences of consuming industrial chemicals whose safety had never been thoroughly tested.

The Soy Discovery

My suspicions proved justified in the most unexpected way. Three years ago, after developing mysterious digestive issues that coincided with a period of taking multiple medications, I worked with my doctors to identify potential triggers. We systematically eliminated foods from my diet, but nothing seemed to help.

Then my physician suggested we look at my medications.

What we discovered shocked both of us: nearly every over-the-counter medication I was taking contained soy as a binding agent, filler, or coating ingredient. The Advil I took for minor aches, the Tums for occasional heartburn, even the multivitamin I'd been swallowing daily for years—all contained various forms of soy protein, soy lecithin, or soy-derived compounds.

This wasn't listed prominently anywhere. You had to dig through the fine print on package inserts, and even then, the soy derivatives were often disguised under chemical names that gave no indication of their origin. "Lecithin" doesn't sound like soy. "Polysorbate 80" doesn't sound like soy. But both can be derived from soybeans, and both were in medications I was taking daily.

When we eliminated all soy-containing medications from my routine, my digestive issues disappeared within two weeks.

The Dairy Revelation

Emboldened by this discovery, we started investigating other common allergens hidden in my medications. The next revelation was even more disturbing: dairy products are everywhere in pharmaceuticals.

Lactose—milk sugar—is one of the most common inactive ingredients in prescription and over-the-counter medications. It's cheap, readily available, and works well as a filler and binding agent. But for the millions of Americans who are lactose intolerant or have dairy allergies, this hidden ingredient can cause everything from digestive distress to severe allergic reactions.

My blood pressure medication contained lactose. My antihistamine contained lactose. Even my supposedly "hypoallergenic" supplements contained dairy-derived compounds. And just like with soy, this information was buried in technical ingredient lists that neither my doctors nor my pharmacists had ever bothered to review with me.

The irony was staggering I was taking antihistamines that contained dairy while trying to figure out why I was having allergic reactions. I was consuming lactose in my digestive medications while wondering why my stomach problems persisted.

The System's Willful Blindness

What became clear through this personal investigation was that our entire medical system operates on a foundation of willful ignorance about pharmaceutical ingredients. Doctors are trained to think about active ingredients and primary effects. They learn to match symptoms with drug categories: pain gets opioids, inflammation gets NSAIDs, infection gets antibiotics.

But they're not trained as chemists or toxicologists. They don't learn about manufacturing processes, contamination risks, or the cumulative effects of consuming multiple chemical additives over time. Most importantly, they're not taught to consider that "inactive" ingredients might be causing active problems for their patients.

The system treats these hidden ingredients as irrelevant background noise, despite the fact that they often make up the majority of what patients are actually swallowing. It's like being served a meal where the chef tells you about the main ingredient while keeping the rest of the recipe secret—and then acting surprised when you have an allergic reaction.

The Trust Trap

Your doctor hands you a prescription. You take it to the pharmacy, receive a bottle of pills, and swallow them without question. This simple act of trust happens millions of times every day across America. We trust our doctors to know what they're prescribing. We trust our pharmacists to dispense what's safe. We trust the FDA to ensure what reaches our medicine cabinets won't harm us.

That trust is killing us.

My decades of surgeries and subsequent medication experiences taught me a harsh truth: your doctor doesn't actually know what's in the medication they just prescribed. The pharmacist filling your prescription has never seen the manufacturing facility where your pills were made. The FDA inspector who "approved" your medication hasn't set foot in the factory that produced it in over three years.

This isn't conspiracy theory. This is the documented reality of modern pharmaceutical manufacturing and medical practice.

The Prescription Assembly Line

Walk into any doctor's office today and witness a system designed for speed, not scrutiny. The average primary care physician sees a patient every 15 minutes. In that quarter-hour, they're expected to diagnose your problem, consider your medical history, weigh potential treatments, and write a prescription. What they're not doing—what they literally don't have time to do—is researching the complete chemical composition of the medication they're about to put into your body.

Your doctor learned about medications in medical school from textbooks that focus on active ingredients and primary effects. They receive continuing education from pharmaceutical sales representatives whose job is to sell drugs, not to exhaustively detail every chemical component and manufacturing risk. They rely on the Physicians' Desk Reference and similar resources that list "active ingredients" prominently while relegating the other 60-80% of each pill's contents to fine print labeled as "inactive ingredients."

But here's the critical truth I learned through my own health struggles: there's no such thing as an inactive ingredient when it comes to your body's chemical reactions.

The Illusion of Regulation

The FDA—the agency we've entrusted with keeping our medications safe—operates under a system of assumptions rather than verification. They assume that pharmaceutical companies are telling the truth about their manufacturing processes. They assume that overseas facilities maintain American standards even when inspected infrequently or never. They assume that "inactive" ingredients that were deemed safe decades ago remain safe when combined with new active compounds, consumed by people taking multiple medications, or manufactured under different conditions than originally tested.

These assumptions are built into the very foundation of drug approval. When a pharmaceutical company submits a new drug application, they're not required to prove that every single chemical component is safe for every potential user in every possible combination. They're required to prove that the active ingredient works for its intended purpose and doesn't cause more harm than benefit in clinical trials that typically last a few months and involve carefully selected participants.

The manufacturing facilities where your medications are actually produced? The FDA inspects domestic facilities on average every two to three years. Foreign facilities—which now produce approximately 80% of the active pharmaceutical ingredients in American medications—are inspected even less frequently. Some have never been inspected at all.

The Chemical Reality

Every pill in your medicine cabinet is a complex chemical cocktail. That innocent-looking white tablet contains not just the medication you think you're taking, but a carefully engineered mixture of binding agents, fillers, preservatives, dyes, coatings, lubricants, and stabilizers. Many of these substances are industrial chemicals that happen to be useful in pharmaceutical manufacturing. Some are known allergens. Others are compounds that have never been tested for long-term human consumption.

The manufacturers aren't hiding this information—it's printed right on the package insert that nobody reads. But they're not advertising it either. When was the last time you saw a drug commercial mention that their antidepressant contains formaldehyde, or that their blood pressure medication includes a plastic coating made from the same polymer used in disposable cups?

These aren't accidents or contamination events. These are intentional ingredients, added because they serve specific manufacturing purposes. The formaldehyde prevents bacterial growth. The plastic coating controls how quickly the drug dissolves. The soy lecithin helps bind the tablet together. The lactose makes the pill the right size and weight.

Your body doesn't distinguish between intentional and accidental chemical exposure—it simply responds to whatever you've put into it. As I learned the hard way, even "inactive" ingredients can trigger continually active health problems.

The Hidden Allergen Crisis

My experience with soy and dairy contamination in medications is not unique—it's epidemic. Millions of Americans with food allergies, intolerances, and sensitivities are unknowingly consuming their trigger substances in their daily medications. The reactions are often attributed to their underlying conditions, side effects of the active ingredients, or mysterious unexplained symptoms.

Corn derivatives are in countless medications, threatening people with corn allergies. Gluten appears in many prescription drugs, potentially harmful to those with celiac disease. Artificial dyes derived from petroleum products are added for cosmetic purposes, despite links to behavioral problems in sensitive individuals. Preservatives that are banned in food products for children are routinely included in children's medications.

The medical system's response to these problems is typically to prescribe additional medications to treat the symptoms caused by the original medications—creating a cascade of chemical exposure that compounds the problem.

The Contamination Crisis

Beyond the intentionally added chemicals lies an even more disturbing reality: widespread contamination that's discovered only after millions of people have consumed affected medications. In recent years, we've seen blood pressure medications contaminated with probable carcinogens, antacids laced with rocket fuel components, and generic drugs tainted with glass particles, metal fragments, and bacterial toxins.

These contamination events aren't rare anomalies—they're the predictable result of a system that prioritizes cost and speed over safety and transparency. When pharmaceutical manufacturing moved overseas to countries with lower labor costs and less stringent oversight, we didn't just export jobs. We exported our ability to ensure the safety of our medication supply.

The Prescription Paradox

Here's the paradox that defines modern medicine: the same doctors who advise you to eat organic food, avoid processed chemicals, and read ingredient labels on everything from shampoo to breakfast cereal will prescribe medications without knowing or discussing the complete chemical content of what they're recommending.

They'll spend twenty minutes explaining the side effects of a medication's active ingredient but won't mention that the pill also contains potential allergens, industrial lubricants, or chemical preservatives. They'll carefully consider drug interactions between active ingredients while ignoring how the dozens of inactive ingredients might interact with each other, with your food, or with your other medications.

This isn't malice or incompetence—it's a system that has evolved to treat doctors as drug distributors rather than chemical safety experts. They're trained to match symptoms with active ingredients, not to serve as toxicologists evaluating the safety of complex chemical mixtures.

The Cost of Ignorance

The consequences of this willful ignorance are measured not just in individual health outcomes, but in the broader erosion of public trust in medicine and regulatory institutions. When people discover that their "FDA-approved" medication was manufactured in facilities that have never been inspected, or that their prescription contains chemicals that were never tested for long-term safety, they lose faith in the entire system.

Some turn to alternative medicine, which often lacks any regulation at all. Others simply stop taking necessary medications, risking their health in a unique way. Many continue taking their prescriptions while harboring growing anxiety about what they're really putting into their bodies.

My own journey led me to become increasingly selective about which medications I was willing to take, often choosing to manage pain and other symptoms through non-pharmaceutical means rather than consuming chemical cocktails I couldn't trust.

Why This Book Matters Now

We stand at a crossroads in pharmaceutical safety. The COVID-19 pandemic highlighted both the incredible potential of modern drug development and the fragility of our global supply chains. Shortages revealed how dependent we've become on overseas manufacturing we can't adequately monitor. Emergency authorizations demonstrated that safety testing can be abbreviated when the stakes are high enough.

The question we must now ask is: if the stakes are always high when it comes to the chemicals we put in our bodies, why do we accept abbreviated safety measures as standard practice?

This book will take you inside the world of pharmaceutical manufacturing, regulatory oversight, and medical practice to show you exactly what's in the medications you and your loved ones take every day. You'll discover how the drugs are really made, where the chemicals come from, and why neither your doctor nor the FDA can guarantee their complete safety.

More importantly, you'll learn how to protect yourself and your family by asking the right questions, demanding better information, and making more informed decisions about the chemical risks you're willing to accept in exchange for medical benefits.

My Eighteen surgeries taught me that questioning your medications isn't paranoia—it's necessary self-preservation. The trust trap has caught millions of Americans who believed that someone else was watching out for their safety. It's time to start watching out for yourself.

Your health—and your life—may depend on what you discover in the pages that follow.

Chapter 1: Beyond the Active Ingredient

What's really in that little pill you just swallowed?

Sarah reached for her morning routine: a multivitamin, her blood pressure medication, and two Tylenol for the headache that had been nagging her since yesterday. Like millions of Americans, she performed this ritual without a second thought, trusting that these small capsules and tablets contained exactly what she needed—nothing more, nothing less. But if Sarah had turned over that bottle of Extra Strength Tylenol and really examined the ingredient list, she might have been surprised to discover that the acetaminophen she thought she was taking made up less than half of what she actually swallowed.

Welcome to the hidden world of pharmaceutical chemistry, where the "medicine" in your medicine cabinet tells only part of the story.

The Great Pharmaceutical Illusion

We live in an age of unprecedented medical transparency. We can look up drug interactions online, read about side effects, and even access clinical trial data with a few clicks. Yet most of us remain completely in the dark about one fundamental question: What exactly are we putting into our bodies when we take medication?

The answer might surprise you. That little white pill isn't just medicine—it's a carefully engineered chemical cocktail containing dozens of ingredients you've probably never heard of. Some of these ingredients help the drug work better. Others help it look prettier, taste better, or last longer on the shelf. Still others are there for reasons that have nothing to do with your health and everything to do with manufacturing efficiency and profit margins.

This isn't a conspiracy theory. It's simply a reality that the pharmaceutical industry hasn't been particularly eager to advertise, and one that most doctors don't think to discuss with their patients. After all, when was the last time your physician explained the difference between the "active ingredient" and the other 15-20 substances in your prescription?

The Myth of "Just Medicine"

Most people operate under what we might call the "pure drug myth"—the assumption that medications contain only the therapeutic substance needed to treat their condition, perhaps with a small amount of harmless filler to hold the pill together. This misconception is so widespread that even many healthcare professionals don't fully grasp the complexity of modern pharmaceutical formulations.

The reality is far more complicated. Every medication is actually a sophisticated delivery system, engineered not just to provide a therapeutic effect, but to meet dozens of other requirements: it must be stable enough to survive months or years on a shelf, attractive enough for patients to willingly swallow, consistent enough to pass regulatory standards, and profitable enough to justify manufacturing costs.

To achieve all of these goals, pharmaceutical companies rely on what the industry calls "excipients"—a clinical term for all the ingredients in a medication that aren't the active drug itself. These excipients aren't just harmless fillers; they're active participants in how your medication works, how your body processes it, and sometimes, how it makes you feel.

The 80/20 Rule: When Medicine Isn't Mostly Medicine

Here's a number that might shock you: in most medications, the actual therapeutic ingredient—the part that's supposed to make you feel better—comprises less than 20% of what you're swallowing. Sometimes it's much less.

Take a standard 500mg Tylenol tablet. The acetaminophen that actually relieves your pain. That's exactly 500mg. But the total weight of the tablet is typically around 850mg. That means more than 40% of what you're ingesting consists of other substances entirely. And that's actually on the conservative side for pharmaceuticals.

Consider birth control pills, where the active hormones might represent less than 1% of the total pill weight. Or extended-release medications, where the actual drug might be buried within layers of polymers, waxes, and release-controlling agents that can make up 80% or more of the final product.

This isn't necessarily problematic—many of these additional ingredients serve crucial functions. But it does mean that when you take a medication, you're not just taking medicine. You're taking a complex mixture of chemicals, each chosen for specific reasons, each with its own properties and potential effects on your body.

Dissecting the Medicine Cabinet: What's Really Inside

Let's take a closer look at some common medications to understand exactly what we're dealing with. We'll start with something almost everyone has taken acetaminophen, commonly known by the brand name Tylenol.

Case Study 1: Extra Strength Tylenol

Pick up a bottle of Extra Strength Tylenol and read the "inactive ingredients" list. Depending on the specific formulation, you might see:

Croscarmellose sodium: A "super disintegrant" that helps the tablet break apart in your stomach

Magnesium stearate: A lubricant that prevents the powder from sticking to manufacturing equipment

Microcrystalline cellulose: A filler that gives the tablet bulk and structure

Polyethylene glycol: A polymer that can affect how quickly the drug dissolves

Povidone: A binding agent that holds the tablet together

Pregelatinized starch: Another disintegrant and filler

Sodium starch glycolate: Yet another disintegrant

Stearic acid: Another lubricant

Titanium dioxide: A whitening agent that makes the pill look clean and uniform

That's nine additional chemicals in addition to the acetaminophen—and this is considered a relatively simple formulation. Each of these ingredients was chosen for specific reasons, but none of them are there to treat your headache.

Some of these substances are generally recognized as safe in the amounts used. Others have sparked debate within the scientific community. Titanium dioxide, for instance, has been banned as a food additive in the European Union due to potential health concerns, yet it remains common in American pharmaceuticals.

Case Study 2: Advil (Ibuprofen)

Let's examine another common pain reliever: Advil. A typical 200mg Advil tablet contains:

Active ingredient:

Ibuprofen: 200mg

Inactive ingredients:

Acetylated monoglycerides: Emulsifiers that help ingredients mix properly

Colloidal silicon dioxide: An anti-caking agent that prevents clumping

Corn starch: A disintegrant and filler

Croscarmellose sodium: The same super disintegrant we saw in Tylenol

Methylparaben: A preservative that prevents bacterial growth

Microcrystalline cellulose: The same filler from Tylenol

Pharmaceutical glaze: A coating that gives the pill its smooth finish

Povidone: The same binding agent from Tylenol

Propylparaben: Another preservative

Silicon dioxide: An anti-caking agent

Sodium benzoate: Yet another preservative

Sodium lauryl sulfate: A surfactant that helps the tablet dissolve

Sodium starch glycolate: The same disintegrant from Tylenol

Stearic acid: The same lubricant from Tylenol

Titanium dioxide: The same whitening agent from Tylenol

That's fifteen additional chemicals beyond the ibuprofen itself. Notice how many ingredients appear in both formulations—this isn't coincidence. The pharmaceutical industry relies on a relatively small palette of well-established excipients, which means if you take multiple medications, you're likely consuming the same additives repeatedly throughout the day.

Case Study 3: Birth Control Pills

Birth control pills represent perhaps the most striking example of the 80/20 rule in action. A typical combination birth control pill contains incredibly lesser amounts of active hormones—we're talking about micrograms, not milligrams.

Take a common brand like Ortho Tri-Cyclen. Each "active" pill contains:

Ethinyl estradiol: 35 micrograms (that's 0.035 milligrams)

Norgestimate: 180-250 micrograms (0.18-0.25 milligrams)

The total weight of active hormones? Less than 0.3 milligrams in most cases. But each pill weighs approximately 100 milligrams. That means more than 99% of what women taking birth control pills swallow every day consists of inactive ingredients.

What makes up the rest? A typical list might include:

Lactose monohydrate: A milk sugar used as a filler

Magnesium stearate: The same lubricant we've seen before

Microcrystalline cellulose: The same filler from pain relievers

Povidone: The same binding agent

Pregelatinized starch: Another filler

FD&C Blue No. 2: Artificial coloring

Hypromellose: A coating agent

Polyethylene glycol: A polymer coating

Titanium dioxide: The same whitening agent

For women with lactose intolerance, the lactose in birth control pills can cause digestive issues—a side effect that has nothing to do with the hormones themselves and everything to do with the "inactive" ingredients.

The Language of Obfuscation

One reason most people don't understand what's in their medications is that the pharmaceutical industry has developed its own language to describe these additives. Terms like "excipients," "pharmaceutical aids," and "inactive ingredients" sound technical and harmless, but they obscure the reality of what these substances actually are and do.

Consider some of the more creative names the industry uses:

What they call "microcrystalline cellulose" is essentially processed wood pulp

"Magnesium stearate" is a salt derived from stearic acid, which often comes from animal fat

"Polyethylene glycol" is closely related to antifreeze (though in much different concentrations)

"Sodium lauryl sulfate" is the same foaming agent found in toothpaste and shampoo

None of this means these ingredients are necessarily dangerous in the amounts used in medications, but it does illustrate how technical terminology can make common substances sound more sophisticated—and less questionable—than they might otherwise appear.

The Regulatory Gray Area

Here's where things get particularly interesting from a regulatory standpoint. While the FDA requires extensive testing and approval for active pharmaceutical ingredients, the oversight of excipients operates under a quite separate set of rules.

Most excipients fall under what the FDA calls "Generally Recognized as Safe" (GRAS) status. This designation often dates back decades and was frequently based on food use rather than pharmaceutical use. The assumption has long been that if something is safe to eat, it's safe to include in a pill.

But this assumption doesn't account for several crucial factors:

Concentration differences: The amount of an excipient in a single pill might be small, but people taking multiple medications daily can accumulate significant quantities of the same additives.

Processing differences: Excipients in pills are often chemically modified versions of food-grade substances, with different properties and potentially different biological effects.

Population differences: Regulatory decisions about excipient safety are typically based on healthy adult populations, not on children, elderly patients, or people with compromised immune systems who might process these chemicals differently.

Interaction effects: While individual excipients might be safe, little research has been done on how they interact with each other or with active pharmaceutical ingredients.

The Manufacturing Imperative

To understand why medications, contain so many non-therapeutic ingredients, it helps to understand the realities of pharmaceutical manufacturing. Modern drug production is a high-volume, high-speed industrial process that prioritizes consistency, efficiency, and shelf stability more than anything else.

Consider the challenges facing a pharmaceutical manufacturer:

Consistency: Every pill must contain exactly the same amount of active ingredient, distributed evenly throughout the tablet. This requires carefully chosen fillers and binding agents.

Manufacturing speed: Production lines might turn out thousands of pills per minute. This requires lubricants to prevent sticking and anti-caking agents to ensure smooth powder flow.

Shelf stability: Pills must remain potent for years under varying storage conditions. This requires preservatives and stabilizers.

Patient compliance: Pills must look, taste, and feel acceptable to patients. This requires colorants, flavorings, and coating agents.

Regulatory compliance: Pills must meet strict standards for hardness, dissolution rate, and appearance. This often requires additional processing aids.

Each of these requirements adds more chemicals to the final product. From a manufacturing standpoint, these additives are essential. From a patient's standpoint, they represent a complex chemical burden that most people never consented to—or even knew they were accepting.

The Cumulative Effect

Perhaps the most concerning aspect of pharmaceutical excipients isn't any single ingredient, but rather the cumulative effect of consuming dozens of these chemicals daily, often for years or decades.

Consider a typical American adult taking what might be considered a modest medication regimen:

A daily multivitamin

A prescription for high blood pressure

An occasional pain reliever

A prescription sleep aids a few times per week

This seemingly simple regimen could easily expose someone to 30-40 different excipients daily, some of them in multiple medications. Over the course of a year, this person might consume several grams of titanium dioxide, magnesium stearate, microcrystalline cellulose, and other additives.

We simply don't have comprehensive data on what this kind of chronic, low-level exposure to multiple chemical additives does to human health over time. The research that does exist focuses on individual ingredients in isolation, not on the complex mixtures that people actually consume.

Questions Your Doctor Probably Can't Answer

This brings us to an uncomfortable truth: most healthcare providers know remarkably little about the non-active ingredients in the medications they prescribe. Medical education focuses intensively on pharmacology—how drugs work in the body—but pays minimal attention to pharmaceutical chemistry and excipient science.

Ask your doctor these questions and see what kind of answers you get:

"What's the total amount of titanium dioxide I'm consuming if I take three different medications that contain it?"

"Could the magnesium stearate in my medications be affecting my magnesium levels?"

"Why does my birth control pill contain lactose when I'm lactose intolerant?"

"Are there versions of my medications that use different excipients?"

"What research has been done on the long-term effects of consuming these additives daily?"

Chances are that your doctor won't have ready answers to these questions. This isn't a failing on their part—it's a reflection of how little emphasis the medical system places on understanding the complete chemical profile of medications.

The International Perspective

It's worth noting that different countries have different standards for pharmaceutical excipients, which raises interesting questions about what's absolutely necessary versus what's simply convenient for manufacturers.

For example:

European medications often use different colorants than American versions of the same drugs

Some countries have banned certain excipients (like certain artificial colors) that remain common in US medications

Generic medications in different countries may use entirely different excipient profiles for the same active ingredient

If a medication works equally well with different excipients in different countries, it raises questions about whether all the additives in American formulations are necessary.

The Path Forward: Becoming an Informed Consumer

The goal of this examination isn't to scare people away from necessary medications. Modern pharmaceuticals have saved countless lives and improved the quality of life for millions of people. Rather, the goal is to encourage a more informed approach to medication use—one that considers the complete chemical picture, not just the active ingredients.

This means:

Reading labels completely: Don't just look at the active ingredients. Read the complete ingredient list and research anything you don't recognize.

Asking better questions: Ask your pharmacist about excipient alternatives. Many medications are available in different formulations with different additive profiles.

Understanding your total exposure: If you take multiple medications, add up your daily exposure to common excipients like titanium dioxide or magnesium stearate.

Considering timing: Some excipients can affect the absorption of nutrients or other medications. Understanding what's in your pills can help you time doses more effectively.

Staying informed: The science around pharmaceutical excipients is evolving. New research occasionally reveals concerns about ingredients that were previously considered completely safe.

The Questions We Should Be Asking

As we move forward in this exploration of pharmaceutical chemistry, several fundamental questions deserve our attention:

Why are we so comfortable consuming dozens of chemical additives daily without understanding what they are or what they do?

Why don't doctors routinely discuss excipients with patients, especially those taking multiple medications?

Why do we accept that most of what we swallow when taking medicine isn't actually medicine?

How do we balance the legitimate manufacturing needs of pharmaceutical companies with patients' right to understand—and consent to—everything they're putting in their bodies?

What would medications look like if they were designed primarily for patient health rather than manufacturing efficiency?

These aren't anti-pharmaceutical questions. They're pro-patient questions. They reflect a desire for transparency, informed consent, and a healthcare system that treats patients as partners rather than passive consumers.

The Hidden Chemical Story Continues

What we've examined so far—the basic ingredients in common medications—represents just the beginning. As we'll see in subsequent chapters, the story of what's really in our drugs extends far beyond simple ingredient lists.

We'll explore how these chemicals interact with each other and with our bodies in ways that aren't fully understood. We'll examine the manufacturing processes that can introduce contaminants and impurities. We'll look at how different populations—children, elderly adults, people with chronic diseases—might be affected differently by the same excipients.

We'll also examine the economic and regulatory forces that shape pharmaceutical formulations, often in ways that prioritize convenience and profit over patient health. And we'll explore alternatives—ways that medications could be formulated differently, and steps that informed patients can take to minimize their exposure to unnecessary chemical additives.

But first, we need to acknowledge a simple truth: when you take a pill, you're not just taking medicine. You're taking a complex chemical mixture that includes the medicine you want, plus a dozen or more other substances that you probably didn't know you were agreeing to consume.

The question isn't whether this is good or bad—it's whether you have the right to know about it, understand it, and make informed decisions based on complete information.

We believe you do.

The journey toward becoming a truly informed pharmaceutical consumer starts with understanding that the pill in your hand contains far more than meets the eye. What you choose to do with that knowledge is up to you.

But first, you need to have the knowledge. And that's exactly what this book aims to provide.

Chapter 2: The Manufacturing Web

The label on your prescription bottle says, "Manufactured by Pfizer, New York" or "Distributed by Johnson & Johnson, New Brunswick, NJ." These familiar American company names provide a comforting sense of domestic quality control and FDA oversight. You assume your medication was made in a state-of-the-art facility somewhere in America, subject to rigorous inspection and quality standards.

You would be wrong.

The reality of modern pharmaceutical manufacturing is a complex global web that would shock most patients—and apparently most doctors—who remain blissfully unaware of where their medications actually originate. That Pfizer label might mean your pills were manufactured in a facility in rural China that hasn't been inspected by the FDA in five years. That Johnson & Johnson product could contain active ingredients sourced from a plant in India that was flagged for safety violations but continues operating while appeals drag through bureaucratic channels.

After my discovery of hidden soy and dairy in medications, I became obsessed with understanding not just what was in my pills, but where they came from and how they were made. What I uncovered was a manufacturing system that prioritizes cost savings over safety, regulatory compliance over actual oversight, and corporate profits over patient protection.

The Great Migration

To understand how we arrived at this precarious situation, we need to go back to the 1990s, when American pharmaceutical companies made a fateful decision that would fundamentally alter the safety of our medication supply. Facing pressure to reduce costs and increase profits, these companies began systematically moving their manufacturing operations overseas to countries with lower labor costs and fewer regulatory restrictions.

It started gradually. First, companies moved the production of basic chemicals and raw materials to countries like India and China, where skilled chemists could be hired for a fraction of American wages. The finished medications, they assured regulators and the public, would still be manufactured in FDA-approved facilities in the United States.

But economic pressures proved irresistible. By the early 2000s, companies were moving not just raw material production, but active pharmaceutical ingredient (API) manufacturing overseas. Then came finished dosage form production—the actual pill-making process. Today, according to the FDA's own estimates, approximately 80% of the active pharmaceutical ingredients in American medications are manufactured outside the United States, with the majority coming from facilities in India and China.

This isn't just about generic medications, though they represent the most extreme example of overseas dependency. Even brand-name drugs from major American pharmaceutical companies rely heavily on foreign manufacturing. When you pick up your prescription for Lipitor, Zoloft, or virtually any other common medication, there's a high probability that critical components were manufactured in facilities thousands of miles away from any meaningful FDA oversight.

The India Phenomenon

India has become the world's pharmacy, producing an estimated 40% of all generic medications consumed in the United States. The country's pharmaceutical industry employs over 3 million people and operates more than 3,000 drug manufacturing facilities. These numbers sound impressive until you realize that the FDA has only about 20 investigators responsible for inspecting facilities across the entire country.

The math is sobering with thousands of facilities and a handful of inspectors, the average Indian pharmaceutical plant can expect an FDA inspection perhaps once every decade, if at all. Many facilities that supply critical medications to American patients have never been inspected by American regulators.

But the problem isn't just the frequency of inspections—it's the quality and reliability of the manufacturing processes in many of these facilities. Over the past decade, the FDA has issued warning letters to hundreds of Indian pharmaceutical companies for violations including:

Falsifying testing data to hide contamination

Using water contaminated with bacteria for medication production

Failing to investigate obvious signs of contamination

Manipulating stability testing to extend expiration dates

Mixing different batches of medications to hide quality problems

In 2019, the FDA banned imports from Ranbaxy Laboratories, one of India's largest generic drug manufacturers, after discovering the company had been systematically falsifying data for years. Medications that had been consumed by millions of Americans were found to contain impurities, incorrect dosages, and contamination that the company had known about but concealed from regulators.

The Ranbaxy case wasn't an isolated incident—it was a window into standard operating procedures at many overseas manufacturing facilities. Internal company documents revealed that executives knew their medications didn't meet safety standards but continued shipping them to American patients while hiding evidence from FDA investigators.

China's Chemical Dominance

While India dominates finished medication production, China has become the primary source of the basic chemical building blocks that go into virtually all medications. An estimated 90% of the active pharmaceutical ingredients used in American medications either come directly from China or rely on Chinese-produced precursor chemicals.

This dependency became dramatically apparent during the early days of the COVID-19 pandemic, when supply chain disruptions in China led to immediate shortages of critical medications in American hospitals. Suddenly, healthcare providers realized that antibiotics, sedatives, and other essential drugs they'd assumed were domestically produced were actually dependent on chemical supplies from factories in Wuhan and other Chinese cities that had been shut down by pandemic lockdowns.

The concentration of pharmaceutical chemical production in China creates multiple vulnerability points:

Single-source dependency: Many critical medications rely on active ingredients produced by just one or two Chinese facilities. If a single factory shuts down due to contamination, regulatory action, or natural disaster, American patients can face immediate shortages of life-saving medications.

Quality control challenges: Chinese pharmaceutical chemical production operates under regulatory standards that differ significantly from American requirements. The FDA's ability to inspect Chinese facilities is even more limited than in India, with language barriers and diplomatic restrictions creating additional obstacles to meaningful oversight.

Environmental contamination: Many Chinese pharmaceutical facilities operate in heavily polluted industrial zones where air and water contamination can directly impact the purity of pharmaceutical products. Medications manufactured in these areas may contain environmental contaminants that would never be detected through standard quality testing.

Regulatory arbitrage: Some Chinese companies specifically target pharmaceutical chemical production because environmental and safety regulations are less strictly enforced than in other industries. This creates a race-to-the-bottom dynamic where the cheapest suppliers often have the worst safety records.

The FDA's Impossible Task

The Food and Drug Administration faces a regulatory challenge that would have been unimaginable when the agency was created: ensuring the safety of medications manufactured in countries where they have limited authority, restricted access, and cultural and language barriers that complicate oversight.

The FDA's Office of Global Policy and Strategy employs approximately 200 investigators responsible for inspecting pharmaceutical facilities worldwide. These investigators must cover over 3,000 foreign facilities across dozens of countries, many in remote locations with limited infrastructure and communication capabilities.

Consider the logistics: An FDA inspector based in the United States receives a tip about potential contamination at a facility in rural India. First, they must obtain approval for the inspection from both American and Indian authorities—a process that can take months. Then they must coordinate travel, interpreters, and local logistics. The inspection itself might last three to five days, during which facility managers have a chance to hide evidence or temporarily modify their procedures.

Even when inspectors identify serious violations, enforcement becomes a diplomatic and legal nightmare. The FDA can ban imports from specific facilities, but companies often simply restructure, rename their operations, or shift production to uninspected facilities. The agency's authority to impose meaningful penalties on foreign manufacturers is severely limited by international law and trade agreements.

The Warning Letter Charade

When FDA inspectors discover violations at overseas facilities, their primary enforcement tool is the warning letter—a formal notification that gives companies an opportunity to correct problems voluntarily. These letters are supposed to be the first step in an escalating enforcement process that can ultimately lead to import bans and criminal prosecution.

In practice, warning letters have become a bureaucratic ritual that allows both regulators and manufacturers to claim they're addressing safety problems while changing little. Companies respond to warning letters with detailed "corrective action plans" that promise to fix identified problems, often without actually implementing meaningful changes.

The FDA's own data reveals the inadequacy of this system: approximately 60% of foreign facilities that receive warning letters for serious violations continue operating without meaningful intervention. Many facilities receive multiple warning letters over several years while continuing to supply medications to American patients.

Case Study: The Heparin Contamination Crisis of 2008

No case better illustrates the dangers of our globalized pharmaceutical supply chain than the heparin contamination crisis that killed at least 81 Americans and sickened hundreds more in 2008. Heparin, a blood-thinning medication essential for surgery and dialysis, had been safely produced for decades using standardized processes and quality controls.

The crisis began when American pharmaceutical companies, seeking to reduce costs, began sourcing heparin from Chinese suppliers who could produce the medication at a fraction of the price charged by domestic manufacturers. The companies assured regulators that the Chinese-produced heparin was identical to the American product and subject to the same quality standards.

They were catastrophically wrong.

The Contamination

In late 2007, patients across the United States began experiencing severe allergic reactions during medical procedures involving heparin. Symptoms included difficulty breathing, rapid heartbeat, severe drop in blood pressure, and in some cases, cardiac arrest. Initially, these reactions were attributed to individual patient sensitivities or unrelated medical complications.

It wasn't until dozens of deaths had occurred that investigators identified the common factor: all victims had received heparin from batches produced by Chinese suppliers. Laboratory analysis revealed that the heparin contained a deliberately added contaminant—over-sulfated chondroitin sulfate (OSCS), a chemically similar but medically dangerous substance that could mimic heparin in basic quality tests while causing severe allergic reactions in patients.

The Cover-Up

The contamination wasn't accidental—it was a deliberate act of economic fraud. Chinese suppliers had been systematically adulterating their heparin with OSCS, a much cheaper substance that could pass standard quality tests while stretching their supplies and increasing profits. The adulteration had been ongoing for months or possibly years before American patients began dying.

Even more disturbing was the discovery that American pharmaceutical companies had failed to conduct adequate quality testing that would have detected the contamination. They had relied on basic tests that verified the presence of heparin-like activity without specifically testing for dangerous adulterants.

The Regulatory Failure

The FDA's investigation revealed a cascade of regulatory failures that had enabled the contamination to reach American patients:

No facility inspections: The Chinese facilities producing the contaminated heparin had never been inspected by FDA investigators, despite supplying critical medications to American hospitals.

Inadequate testing requirements: The quality standards for heparin didn't require specific testing for OSCS or other potential adulterants that could cause the observed reactions.

Supply chain opacity: American pharmaceutical companies couldn't trace their heparin supplies back to the original source facilities, making it impossible to quickly identify and isolate contaminated batches.

Delayed response: The FDA didn't issue a public warning about the contamination until months after the first deaths had occurred, allowing contaminated heparin to continue reaching patients.

The Aftermath

The heparin crisis led to immediate changes in how the FDA approaches overseas pharmaceutical manufacturing, but these reforms have proved largely inadequate. The agency increased inspection frequency for critical medication suppliers and enhanced testing requirements for heparin specifically. However, the fundamental problems that enabled the crisis—limited oversight of foreign facilities, inadequate quality testing, and supply chain opacity—remain largely unchanged.

More troubling, internal FDA documents obtained through Freedom of Information Act requests reveal that agency officials knew about quality problems at Chinese pharmaceutical facilities years before the heparin crisis but failed to take meaningful action. Warning letters had been sent to multiple Chinese heparin suppliers documenting serious quality control violations, but imports continued without interruption.

The Ongoing Crisis

The heparin contamination crisis was a watershed moment that should have fundamentally reformed pharmaceutical manufacturing oversight. Instead, it has become a case study in how regulatory agencies and pharmaceutical companies can acknowledge serious safety problems while implementing only cosmetic changes that fail to address underlying systemic issues.

Today, more than fifteen years after the crisis, American patients remain dependent on medications manufactured in overseas facilities with minimal oversight. The FDA continues to rely primarily on warning letters and voluntary compliance to address safety violations at foreign manufacturers. Supply chain transparency has improved marginally, but most patients and even most doctors still have no idea where their medications are actually produced.

Recent Contamination Events

The problems haven't stopped with heparin. In recent years, we've seen:

Valsartan contamination (2018-2019): Blood pressure medications contaminated with probable carcinogens, affecting millions of patients and leading to one of the largest drug recalls in history.

Ranitidine contamination (2019-2020): The popular heartburn medication Zantac was found to contain NDMA, a probable carcinogen, leading to its complete removal from the American market.

Metformin contamination (2020-2021): The diabetes medication was found to contain excessive levels of NDMA in products manufactured by multiple overseas suppliers.

Each of these contamination events followed the same pattern: overseas manufacturing facilities cutting corners on safety, inadequate quality testing by American pharmaceutical companies, delayed detection by regulatory agencies, and belated warnings to patients after potentially harmful exposure had already occurred.

The Economic Reality

The pharmaceutical industry's defense of overseas manufacturing typically focuses on cost savings that supposedly benefit consumers through lower medication prices. This argument conveniently ignores several inconvenient realities:

Cost savings don't reach patients: While pharmaceutical companies have dramatically reduced their manufacturing costs by moving production overseas, prescription drug prices in the United States have continued to rise faster than inflation. The savings from overseas manufacturing have been captured by pharmaceutical companies and their shareholders, not passed on to patients.

Hidden costs of contamination: The direct costs of medication recall, patient treatment for contamination-related illnesses, and regulatory enforcement actions are ultimately borne by patients and taxpayers, not pharmaceutical companies. These hidden costs often exceed any savings from cheaper manufacturing.

National security vulnerabilities: The concentration of pharmaceutical manufacturing in potentially hostile foreign countries creates national security risks that carry costs beyond simple economics. During international crises or conflicts, American patients could face immediate shortages of critical medications.

Innovation disincentives: Moving manufacturing overseas often means moving pharmaceutical expertise and innovation capacity as well. American pharmaceutical companies increasingly rely on foreign partners not just for manufacturing, but for process development and quality improvement.

The Supply Chain Shell Game

Perhaps the most frustrating aspect of investigating pharmaceutical supply chains is the deliberate opacity that makes it nearly impossible for patients, doctors, or even regulators to trace medications back to their actual manufacturing sources. Pharmaceutical companies have created complex networks of subsidiaries, contractors, and distributors that obscure the true origins of their products.

A typical generic medication might follow this path:

Raw materials sourced from chemical companies in China

Active pharmaceutical ingredients processed at facilities in India owned by subsidiaries of American companies

Finished medications produced at contract manufacturing facilities operated by third-party companies

Packaging and labeling completed at different facilities, often in different countries

Distribution through multiple wholesalers before reaching American pharmacies

At each step in this process, responsibility for quality control and safety becomes more diffuse. When contamination occurs, it can take months to trace products back to their source, during which time patients continue consuming potentially dangerous medications.

The pharmaceutical industry argues that this complexity is necessary for efficiency and cost control. Critics point out that it also provides perfect cover for avoiding accountability when things go wrong.

What Your Doctor Doesn't Know

The globalization of pharmaceutical manufacturing has created an information gap that affects every aspect of medical practice. When your doctor prescribes a medication, they typically know:

The active ingredient and its expected effects

Common side effects and contraindications

Dosing guidelines and administration instructions

What they almost certainly don't know:

Where the medication was actually manufactured

What inactive ingredients it contains beyond basic categories

Whether the manufacturing facility has a history of quality problems

How recently the facility was inspected by regulators

Whether the medication has been subject to recent recalls or safety alerts

This information gap isn't the result of physician negligence—it's a systemic problem created by pharmaceutical companies and regulatory agencies that treat supply chain details as proprietary information rather than essential safety data.

Medical schools don't teach future doctors how to evaluate pharmaceutical supply chains or manufacturing quality. Continuing education programs focus on clinical effects and patient management, not on the industrial processes that create the medications doctors prescribe daily. Electronic prescribing systems and pharmaceutical databases provide no information about manufacturing origins or quality histories.

The result is a medical system where the people responsible for prescribing medications to patients have no meaningful way to evaluate the safety and quality of the products they're recommending.

The Path Forward

The pharmaceutical manufacturing crisis requires solutions that address both immediate safety concerns and long-term systemic problems. Some potential approaches include:

Supply chain transparency requirements: Pharmaceutical companies should be required to disclose the complete manufacturing chain for their products, including all facilities involved in production, testing, and packaging.

Enhanced inspection authority: The FDA needs expanded authority and resources to conduct meaningful oversight of foreign pharmaceutical facilities, including the ability to impose immediate import bans for facilities that refuse inspection or fail to correct violations.

Domestic manufacturing incentives: Government policies should encourage the return of critical pharmaceutical manufacturing to the United States through tax incentives, grants, and procurement preferences for domestically produced medications.

Patient information systems: Doctors and patients should have access to databases that provide real-time information about medication sources, recall histories, and quality problems.

Alternative supply requirements: For critical medications, pharmaceutical companies should be required to maintain manufacturing capacity in multiple countries to prevent single-source dependency.

The current system treats pharmaceutical manufacturing as just another global commodity business, optimized for cost reduction rather than safety and reliability. Until we recognize that medications are fundamentally different from other consumer products—because contamination can kill rather than just inconvenience—we will continue to see preventable crises that harm patients while enriching pharmaceutical companies.

The next time you pick up a prescription, remember that the pill in your hand may have traveled thousands of miles through facilities that have never been inspected, using processes that prioritize cost over safety, before reaching your medicine cabinet. The manufacturing web that produces our medications is vast, complex, and largely invisible—but its consequences for your health are very real.

Chapter 3: Regulatory Blind Spots

When I started questioning what was really in my medications, I assumed the FDA had rigorously tested every component before approving them for human consumption. After all, this is the same agency that requires years of clinical trials for new drugs, monitors adverse events, and has the authority to recall dangerous products from the market. Surely, I thought, they must know exactly what's in every pill and have verified its safety.

I couldn't have been more wrong.

What I discovered through months of research into FDA regulations and approval processes is a system built on assumptions, shortcuts, and regulatory blind spots that would shock anyone who believes government agencies are protecting them from chemical harm. The FDA's approach to medication safety is like a security system that carefully guards the front door while leaving every window and back entrance wide open.

The reality is that the vast majority of chemicals in your medications have never been specifically tested for safety by the FDA. Instead, they operate under a patchwork of assumptions, grandfather clauses, and loopholes that allow pharmaceutical companies to include virtually any substance they want, as long as it serves a manufacturing purpose and isn't immediately toxic in large doses.

How FDA Approval Actually Works

Most people imagine the FDA approval process as a comprehensive evaluation where scientists test every aspect of a medication for safety and effectiveness. The reality is far more limited and focused than this idealized version suggests.

When a pharmaceutical company seeks approval for a new medication, they must demonstrate two primary things: that the active ingredient is effective for its intended use, and that the overall product doesn't cause more harm than benefit in the populations studied. Notice what's missing from this requirement—any specific evaluation of the safety of inactive ingredients, manufacturing chemicals, or long-term cumulative effects of consuming multiple pharmaceutical additives.

The FDA's review process focuses almost entirely on the active pharmaceutical ingredient (API)—the part of the pill that's supposed to treat your condition. Clinical trials test whether this active ingredient works and document its side effects when consumed by carefully selected study participants over relatively short periods, typically a few months to a few years.

What Gets Tested:

The active ingredient's effectiveness for specific conditions

Short-term side effects in healthy volunteers and selected patient populations

Interactions between the active ingredient and a limited number of other common medications

Basic toxicity testing to ensure the active ingredient won't cause immediate harm

Stability testing to determine how long the active ingredient remains potent

What Doesn't Get Tested:

The safety of inactive ingredients beyond basic toxicity screens

Long-term effects of consuming pharmaceutical additives over years or decades

Cumulative effects of multiple inactive ingredients consumed across different medications

Interactions between inactive ingredients and other chemicals in patients' bodies

The safety of manufacturing residues and contamination that falls below "acceptable" limits

Effects on vulnerable populations like children, elderly, or those with compromised immune systems

This testing gap creates a fundamental paradox: the FDA knows more about the safety of the smallest component of your medication (the active ingredient, often 10-20% of the pill) than about the largest components (the inactive ingredients that make up 60-80% of what you're swallowing).

The GRAS Loophole

Perhaps the most significant blind spot in pharmaceutical regulation is the "Generally Recognized as Safe" (GRAS) designation, a regulatory shortcut that allows pharmaceutical companies to include virtually any substance in medications without specific safety testing, as long as that substance has been used in other industries or applications.

The GRAS system was originally created for food additives, based on the reasonable assumption that substances with a long history of safe use in food wouldn't require extensive new testing every time they were used in a different food product. The logic was simple: if people had been safely consuming a substance for decades, it was probably safe to continue using it.

Pharmaceutical companies quickly realized they could exploit this system by arguing that any substance used safely in food, cosmetics, or other consumer products should automatically be considered safe for use in medications. This created a massive loophole that allows pharmaceutical manufacturers to include hundreds of chemicals in medications without any specific testing for pharmaceutical applications.

How GRAS Works in Practice:

A pharmaceutical company wants to use a new binding agent in their tablets. Instead of conducting expensive safety studies specific to pharmaceutical use, they simply point to the fact that the same chemical has been used safely in food packaging for twenty years. The FDA accepts this as evidence of safety and allows the chemical to be used in medications without further testing.

The problems with this approach are numerous and serious:

Different exposure patterns: Consuming a substance occasionally in food is quite different from taking it daily in concentrated form as part of a medication regimen. Many substances that are safe in small, occasional doses can become harmful when consumed regularly over months or years.

Different chemical interactions: Chemicals that are safe when consumed with food may interact differently when consumed with active pharmaceutical ingredients or other medication components.

Different user populations: Food additives are generally consumed by healthy people of all ages in varying amounts. Medications are often taken by sick people whose bodies may process chemicals differently, and dosing is much more standardized and concentrated.

Different regulatory oversight: Food additives are subject to ongoing monitoring and can be quickly removed from the market if problems emerge. Pharmaceutical inactive ingredients receive virtually no post-market surveillance once they're approved for use.

The Grandfather Problem

Even more troubling than the GRAS loophole is the pharmaceutical industry's reliance on "grandfathered" ingredients—substances that were approved for use in medications decades ago under safety standards that would be considered woefully inadequate by today's standards.

Many of the most common inactive ingredients in modern medications were approved for pharmaceutical use in the 1950s, 1960s, and 1970s, when our understanding of chemical toxicity, drug interactions, and long-term health effects was primitive compared to current knowledge. These substances were deemed safe based on limited testing that often involved only acute toxicity studies—essentially determining whether they would kill test animals immediately in high doses.

The grandfathering process works like this:

A chemical was approved for pharmaceutical use in 1965 based on safety testing that would be considered inadequate today

That chemical continues to be used in medications simply because it was previously approved

No additional safety testing is required, even as our understanding of chemical toxicity advances

The chemical remains "safe" by regulatory definition, regardless of new scientific evidence that might suggest problems

This system has created a pharmaceutical ingredient list that's essentially frozen in time, based on the limited scientific knowledge and regulatory standards of previous decades. Many substances that are now known to be problematic—or that would never be approved under current testing standards—continue to be used in medications simply because they were approved in an earlier era.

Examples of grandfathered ingredients that would face scrutiny today:

Formaldehyde-releasing preservatives: Many medications contain preservatives that slowly release formaldehyde to prevent bacterial growth. While formaldehyde is now recognized as a probable carcinogen by multiple health agencies, these preservatives remain widely used in medications because they were approved before the carcinogenic potential was understood.

Heavy metal catalysts: Some pharmaceutical manufacturing processes use heavy metal catalysts that can leave trace residues in finished medications. Many of these processes were approved decades ago when the health effects of chronic heavy metal exposure were poorly understood.

Industrial solvents: Various solvents used in pharmaceutical manufacturing and included as inactive ingredients were approved based on industrial safety standards rather than standards appropriate for daily human consumption over extended periods.

What Gets Assumed Safe

The FDA's approach to pharmaceutical regulation relies heavily on assumptions about safety that may or may not reflect reality. These assumptions create regulatory blind spots that pharmaceutical companies can exploit to include questionable substances in medications without triggering additional safety requirements.

Assumption #1: Small doses are always safe The FDA operates under the assumption that any substance that doesn't cause immediate harm in small doses is safe for long-term consumption. This ignores growing scientific understanding of how chemicals can accumulate in the body over time and cause problems through chronic exposure rather than acute toxicity.

Assumption #2: Individual ingredients are safe when combined Regulatory testing typically evaluates individual ingredients in isolation, then assumes they'll be safe when combined with dozens of other chemicals in a finished medication. This ignores the possibility of synergistic effects where chemicals that are individually safe become problematic when consumed together.

Assumption #3: Manufacturing residues below "acceptable" limits are harmless The FDA allows certain levels of contamination and manufacturing residues in medications, based on assumptions about what constitutes "acceptable" exposure. These limits are often based on industrial safety standards rather than standards appropriate for daily consumption by sick people taking multiple medications.

Assumption #4: Historical use equals safety the regulatory system assumes that any chemical with a history of use in pharmaceuticals is safe to continue using, regardless of advances in scientific understanding or changes in exposure patterns.

Assumption #5: One-size-fits-all safety standards FDA safety standards typically assume an average healthy adult consumer and don't account for increased vulnerability in children, elderly patients, people with compromised immune systems, or those taking multiple medications simultaneously.

International Regulatory Differences

One of the most revealing ways to understand the limitations of FDA regulation is to compare American pharmaceutical standards with those used in other developed countries. These comparisons reveal that many substances routinely used in American medications are banned or restricted in countries with more stringent regulatory approaches.

European Union Standards

The European Medicines Agency (EMA) takes a significantly more precautionary approach to pharmaceutical regulation than the FDA. European regulations:

Require specific safety testing for inactive ingredients, not just active compounds

Ban or restrict many artificial colors and preservatives that are commonly used in American medications

Require pharmaceutical companies to demonstrate that inactive ingredients are necessary for the medication's function, not just that they're not immediately harmful

Apply stricter limits on heavy metal contamination and solvent residues

Require more extensive testing for potential interactions between inactive ingredients

Examples of substances banned in European medications but allowed in American ones:

Artificial dye Red #3: This petroleum-derived coloring agent is banned in European medications due to concerns about links to hyperactivity in children and potential carcinogenic effects. It remains widely used in American medications, including children's formulations.

Sodium benzoate in combination with vitamin C: European regulators restrict this combination because it can form benzene, a known carcinogen, under certain conditions. American medications routinely include both substances without restriction.

Certain parabens: Several paraben preservatives that are banned in European medications due to concerns about hormone disruption continue to be used in American pharmaceutical products.

Japanese Standards

Japan's pharmaceutical regulatory system includes several safety requirements that don't exist in American regulation:

Mandatory testing for inactive ingredient interactions with traditional medicines that many Japanese patients use alongside conventional medications

Stricter limits on bacterial contamination in manufacturing facilities

Required disclosure of all manufacturing chemicals, including those used in processing but not present in the final product

More frequent inspection of foreign manufacturing facilities

Canadian Differences

Even Canada, with a regulatory system similar to the United States, includes several additional safety requirements:

Mandatory reporting of all adverse events potentially related to inactive ingredients

Stricter labeling requirements for common allergens in medications

Enhanced quality control standards for generic medications

More restrictive limits on certain heavy metal contaminants

The Enforcement Gap

Even when the FDA does identify problems with pharmaceutical ingredients or manufacturing processes, the agency's enforcement mechanisms are often inadequate to ensure meaningful compliance. The regulatory system relies heavily on voluntary compliance and industry self-reporting, creating opportunities for pharmaceutical companies to continue using problematic ingredients while appearing to cooperate with regulators.

Warning Letter Theater

The FDA's primary enforcement tool for pharmaceutical violations is the warning letter—a formal notification that identifies problems and requests corrective action. These letters are supposed to be the first step in an escalating enforcement process that can ultimately include import bans, facility shutdowns, and criminal prosecution.

In practice, warning letters have become a regulatory ritual that allows both companies and regulators to claim they're addressing safety problems without implementing meaningful changes.

Companies typically respond with detailed "corrective action plans" that promise to fix identified problems, often without actually changing their practices in substantive ways.

FDA data shows that approximately 40% of pharmaceutical facilities that receive warning letters for significant violations continue operating without meaningful intervention. Many facilities receive multiple warning letters over several years while continuing to supply ingredients and finished medications to American patients.

Limited Recall Authority

While the FDA has the authority to order recalls of dangerous medications, the agency rarely exercises this power for problems related to inactive ingredients or manufacturing quality issues. Most pharmaceutical recalls are "voluntary"—meaning companies agree to remove products from the market in cooperation with the FDA rather than under direct regulatory order.

This voluntary approach creates opportunities for pharmaceutical companies to delay recalls, limit their scope, or implement them in ways that minimize fiscal impact rather than maximize patient safety. Companies often negotiate the terms of recalls with the FDA, leading to compromises that may not adequately protect patients.

The Testing We Need vs. The Testing We Get

The regulatory blind spots in pharmaceutical oversight become most apparent when you compare what kind of testing would be necessary to ensure medication safety with what actually gets done under current FDA requirements.

Testing We Need:

Long-term studies of inactive ingredient safety over periods of years or decades

Interaction studies between inactive ingredients and active compounds

Population-specific safety studies for children, elderly, and people with compromised health

Cumulative exposure assessments for people taking multiple medications

Regular monitoring of manufacturing facilities and supply chains

Post-market surveillance for problems related to inactive ingredients

Comprehensive testing for contamination and manufacturing residues

Testing We Get:

Basic toxicity testing for active ingredients only

Short-term clinical trials lasting months, not years

Limited testing for drug interactions between active ingredients

Minimal oversight of inactive ingredient safety

Infrequent inspection of manufacturing facilities

Little to no post-market monitoring of inactive ingredient problems

Acceptance of "generally recognized as safe" designations without pharmaceutical-specific testing

The Cost of Regulatory Gaps

The human cost of the FDA's regulatory blind spots is difficult to quantify precisely because the agency doesn't systematically track health problems related to inactive ingredients. However, the available evidence suggests that these gaps are causing actual harm to American patients.

Consider these documented examples:

Allergen-related reactions: Thousands of patients each year experience allergic reactions to hidden ingredients in their medications, including reactions to lactose, gluten, soy, and artificial dyes. Many of these reactions are misattributed to the active ingredients or underlying health conditions.

Cumulative toxicity: Patients taking multiple medications may be consuming concerning levels of preservatives, heavy metals, and industrial chemicals without any evaluation of cumulative exposure risks.

Manufacturing contamination: The regular discovery of contaminated medications suggests that current oversight of manufacturing processes is inadequate to protect patients from preventable exposure to harmful substances.

Vulnerable population effects: Children, elderly patients, and those with compromised immune systems may be at higher risk from pharmaceutical additives that haven't been specifically tested in these populations.

Reforming the System

Addressing the FDA's regulatory blind spots would require fundamental changes to how pharmaceutical safety is evaluated and monitored. Some necessary reforms include:

Comprehensive ingredient testing: All ingredients in medications, including inactive components, should be subject to safety testing appropriate for their intended use and exposure patterns.

Post-market surveillance: The FDA should systematically monitor for health problems related to inactive ingredients and manufacturing quality issues.

Cumulative exposure assessment: Regulators should evaluate the safety of consuming multiple pharmaceutical additives simultaneously over extended periods.

Vulnerable population protection: Safety standards should specifically account for increased risks in children, elderly patients, and those with compromised health.

International harmonization: American pharmaceutical standards should be aligned with the most protective international standards rather than the most permissive.

Manufacturing oversight: Inspection and quality control of pharmaceutical manufacturing should be frequent, thorough, and mandatory rather than voluntary.

The current regulatory system treats pharmaceutical safety as a problem that can be solved through limited testing of active ingredients while ignoring the complex chemical reality of modern medications. Until we acknowledge that every component of a medication poses potential risks that deserve evaluation, patients will continue to serve as unwitting test subjects for combinations of chemicals that have never been proven safe for long-term human consumption.

The Revolving Door Problem

One of the most troubling aspects of the FDA's regulatory blind spots is how they're perpetuated by the revolving door between the pharmaceutical industry and the regulatory agencies supposed to oversee it. Former FDA officials routinely take high-paying jobs with pharmaceutical companies, while industry executives move into key regulatory positions, creating conflicts of interest that influence how safety standards are developed and enforced.

This revolving door creates a regulatory culture where challenging industry practices or demanding more rigorous testing can be career-limiting for FDA officials who hope to eventually work in the private sector. The result is a regulatory environment that tends to favor industry-friendly interpretations of safety requirements and gives pharmaceutical companies the benefit of the doubt in borderline cases.

Industry Influence on Safety Standards

The pharmaceutical industry plays a direct role in developing many of the safety standards that the FDA uses to evaluate medications. Industry trade groups regularly submit comments on proposed regulations, and pharmaceutical companies fund much of the research that forms the scientific basis for regulatory decisions.

This industry involvement in standard-setting creates inherent conflicts of interest. Companies have obvious financial incentives to promote regulatory approaches that minimize testing requirements and maximize flexibility in ingredient selection.

When the same companies that profit from loose regulatory standards also help write those standards, patient safety inevitably takes a back seat to corporate interests.

Consider the development of contamination limits for pharmaceutical manufacturing. Rather than setting these limits based on what would be ideal for patient safety, the FDA often sets them based on what the industry claims is "technically feasible" or "economically practical." This approach essentially allows pharmaceutical companies to define their own safety requirements based on their manufacturing capabilities and cost considerations.

The Data Suppression Problem

Another critical blind spot in pharmaceutical regulation is the systematic suppression of safety data that might challenge the safety assumptions underlying current regulatory approaches. Pharmaceutical companies routinely conduct internal safety studies that never become exposed, and researchers who discover problems with pharmaceutical ingredients often face pressure to suppress or minimize their findings.

The FDA's own scientists have reported instances where agency leadership suppressed or altered their safety assessments to make them more favorable to pharmaceutical industry interests. Internal FDA documents obtained through Freedom of Information Act requests have revealed cases where scientists recommended against approving certain ingredients or manufacturing processes, only to have their recommendations overruled by agency administrators.

The Academic Research Gap

Independent academic research on pharmaceutical ingredient safety is severely limited by several factors that benefit the pharmaceutical industry. First, most universities don't have the resources to conduct the kind of long-term, large-scale studies that would be necessary to identify safety problems with inactive ingredients. Second, pharmaceutical companies control access to many of the materials and data that would be necessary for independent research.

Most troubling, pharmaceutical companies often use intellectual property claims and trade secret protections to prevent researchers from studying the safety of their products. When academic researchers try to investigate potential problems with pharmaceutical ingredients, they often find themselves blocked by legal barriers that pharmaceutical companies have erected to protect their commercial interests.

This research suppression means that many potential safety problems with pharmaceutical ingredients simply never get studied by independent researchers who don't have financial conflicts of interest.

The Patient Advocacy Failure

Patient advocacy groups, which should serve as a counterbalance to pharmaceutical industry influence, have largely failed to address the problems with inactive ingredient safety. Many of the most prominent patient advocacy organizations receive significant funding from pharmaceutical companies, creating conflicts of interest that limit their willingness to challenge industry practices.

These advocacy groups typically focus on ensuring patient access to medications and supporting research into new treatments, rather than questioning the safety of existing pharmaceutical ingredients and manufacturing processes. When they do address safety issues, they tend to focus on problems with active ingredients rather than the broader chemical safety issues that affect all medications.

The result is that patients have few independent advocates pushing for stronger safety standards and more rigorous testing of pharmaceutical ingredients. The voices calling for better regulation are often drowned out by well-funded industry lobbying and patient advocacy groups that have been co-opted by pharmaceutical industry funding.

International Pressure and Trade Considerations

The FDA's regulatory blind spots are often perpetuated by international trade considerations that prioritize commercial interests over public health. Trade agreements and diplomatic pressure from countries where pharmaceutical manufacturing is concentrated can influence how aggressively the FDA enforces safety standards.

For example, aggressive inspection and enforcement actions against overseas pharmaceutical facilities can trigger diplomatic complaints and threats of trade retaliation. This creates pressure on FDA officials to avoid enforcement actions that might disrupt pharmaceutical supply chains or anger important trading partners.

Similarly, efforts to strengthen safety standards for pharmaceutical ingredients can be challenged as trade barriers if they disadvantage overseas manufacturers. Pharmaceutical companies often argue that more rigorous safety requirements would violate international trade agreements and harm American consumers by increasing costs or limiting access to medications.

The Innovation Excuse

Pharmaceutical companies and their regulatory allies often defend current safety standards by arguing that more rigorous testing requirements would stifle innovation and delay the development of new medications. This argument is used to justify virtually any regulatory shortcut or safety compromise, regardless of the potential risks to patients.

The innovation excuse is particularly pernicious because it frames patient safety and medical progress as competing interests, when in reality they should be complementary goals. Truly innovative pharmaceutical development should include innovative approaches to safety testing and quality control, not shortcuts that expose patients to unnecessary risks.

More importantly, the innovation argument ignores the fact that many of the regulatory blind spots we've discussed have nothing to do with innovation and everything to do with protecting established industry practices that prioritize cost savings over safety.

Looking Forward: The Price of Inaction

The FDA's regulatory blind spots represent a ticking time bomb for American healthcare. As more patients take multiple medications for longer periods, the cumulative risks from untested pharmaceutical ingredients will inevitably manifest in ways that our current regulatory system is unprepared to detect or address.

The heparin contamination crisis, the valsartan recalls, and other recent pharmaceutical safety disasters provide a preview of what we can expect if these regulatory gaps aren't addressed. Each crisis follows the same pattern: regulatory blind spots allow dangerous practices to continue unchecked until a catastrophic failure forces temporary reforms that fail to address underlying systemic problems.

The human cost of maintaining these regulatory blind spots far exceeds any short-term benefits from reduced testing requirements or faster approval processes. When pharmaceutical ingredients that have never been rigorously tested for safety cause cancer, organ damage, or other serious health problems years or decades after exposure, the medical and economic costs dwarf any savings from abbreviated safety evaluation.

When you take your next prescription medication, remember that the FDA has likely tested only a small fraction of what you're putting into your body. The rest is operating under assumptions, grandfather clauses, and regulatory shortcuts that prioritize pharmaceutical industry convenience over patient safety. In a rational system, the burden of proof would be on manufacturers to demonstrate the safety of every component they include in medications. Instead, the burden falls on patients to hope that decades-old assumptions about chemical safety still hold true in today's world of complex drug regimens and chronic medication use.

Chapter 4: The Inactive Ingredient Myth

The term "inactive ingredient" is perhaps the most misleading phrase in all of pharmaceutical marketing. It suggests that these substances are inert—mere packaging material that safely carries the real medicine to your body without causing any effects of their own. This linguistic sleight of hand has convinced millions of patients, and apparently most doctors, that 60-80% of what they're consuming in their daily medications is essentially harmless filler.

After discovering that soy and dairy were hiding in my medications under the guise of "inactive ingredients," I became obsessed with understanding what these substances actually do in your body. What I found demolished any notion that these ingredients are truly inactive. Many of them are biologically active compounds that can trigger allergic reactions, interfere with medication absorption, cause digestive problems, and interact with other chemicals in ways that no one has bothered to study comprehensively.

The pharmaceutical industry's use of the term "inactive" is technically accurate only in the narrowest sense—these ingredients don't contribute to the medication's primary therapeutic effect. But calling them inactive is like calling the engine oil in your car inactive because it doesn't directly power the wheels. These substances perform critical functions that make modern pharmaceutical manufacturing possible, and they interact with your body in complex ways that can significantly impact your health.

The Manufacturing Reality

To understand why medications, contain so many supposedly inactive ingredients, you need to understand the industrial processes used to manufacture modern pharmaceuticals. Creating a pill isn't simply a matter of compressing the active ingredient into tablet form—it's a complex engineering challenge that requires dozens of specialized chemicals to make the process work reliably at mass production scales.

The Basic Challenges:

Most active pharmaceutical ingredients exist as fine powders that are difficult to work with using industrial equipment. They may not compress well into tablets, might be unstable when exposed to air or moisture, could have unpleasant tastes or colors, or may dissolve too quickly or slowly when consumed. The pharmaceutical manufacturing process must solve all these problems while producing millions of identical doses cost-effectively.

The solution is to combine the active ingredient with a carefully designed mixture of excipients—substances that modify the physical, chemical, and biological properties of the medication to make it manufacturable, stable, and effective. These excipients aren't passengers along for the ride; they're essential components that determine how the medication behaves in your body.

Fillers: The Bulk of Your Pill

Fillers, also called diluents, typically make up the largest portion of most medications by weight. Their primary purpose is to provide sufficient bulk to create tablets of a practical size for manufacturing and patient use. Without fillers, most medication tablets would be too small to handle reliably or might be so tiny they'd be impossible to see or swallow safely.

Common Fillers and Their Properties:

Lactose (milk sugar): The most widely used pharmaceutical filler, lactose is cheap, readily available, and has excellent compression properties that make it ideal for high-speed tablet manufacturing. It's also relatively stable and doesn't interact chemically with most active ingredients.

However, lactose is a major allergen that affects millions of Americans with lactose intolerance. When these patients consume lactose-containing medications, they can experience digestive symptoms including bloating, gas, diarrhea, and cramping that are often misattributed to side effects of the active ingredient or the underlying condition being treated.

Microcrystalline cellulose: Derived from wood pulp, this plant-based filler is increasingly used as an alternative to lactose. While generally well-tolerated, it can cause digestive issues in some patients and may interfere with the absorption of certain medications.

Mannitol: A sugar alcohol used as a filler, particularly in chewable tablets and medications designed to dissolve quickly. Mannitol can have a laxative effect when consumed in significant quantities, which can be problematic for patients taking multiple medications containing this filler.

Starch: Various forms of starch from corn, wheat, or potatoes are used as fillers. These can be problematic for patients with specific grain allergies or celiac disease, particularly when the starch source isn't clearly identified on labeling.

The Hidden Problem:

Patients taking multiple medications may consume substantial amounts of these fillers daily without realizing it. Someone taking five different prescription medications might consume several grams of lactose, cellulose, or other fillers each day—enough to cause symptoms in sensitive individuals.

Binders: Holding It All Together

Binders are substances that help hold tablet ingredients together during the compression process and ensure the finished tablet maintains its structural integrity. Without effective binders, tablets would crumble or break apart, making accurate dosing impossible.

Common Binders:

Polyvinylpyrrolidone (PVP): A synthetic polymer widely used in pharmaceutical manufacturing. While generally considered safe, PVP can accumulate in body tissues over time and has been associated with respiratory problems in some individuals.

Hydroxypropyl methylcellulose (HPMC): A chemically modified form of cellulose that provides excellent binding properties. Some patients experience allergic reactions to HPMC, including skin rashes and digestive symptoms.

Gelatin: Derived from animal collagen, gelatin is used in both tablet binding and capsule manufacturing. This ingredient is problematic for vegetarians, vegans, and people with religious dietary restrictions, as well as those with specific animal protein allergies.

Sodium carboxymethylcellulose: A chemically modified cellulose that can cause sodium intake concerns for patients on low-sodium diets and may interact with certain medications that affect electrolyte balance.

Disintegrants: Controlled Destruction

Disintegrants perform the seemingly contradictory function of helping tablets break apart at precisely the right time and location in your digestive system. These substances remain stable during manufacturing and storage but rapidly swell or dissolve when exposed to moisture in your stomach or intestines.

Common Disintegrants:

Croscarmellose sodium: A modified cellulose that rapidly absorbs water and swells, causing tablets to break apart. The sodium content can be significant for patients taking multiple medications, potentially affecting blood pressure and cardiovascular health.

Sodium starch glycolate: Another rapidly swelling disintegrant that can contribute substantial sodium to patients' daily intake. Like other starch-based ingredients, it may be problematic for patients with specific grain allergies.

Crospovidone: A cross-linked form of PVP that provides excellent disintegration properties but shares the potential accumulation concerns associated with other PVP compounds.

Lubricants: Preventing Industrial Friction

Lubricants are added to prevent pharmaceutical ingredients from sticking to manufacturing equipment during the tablet compression process. These substances must reduce friction between the tablet mixture and metal surfaces while not interfering with the medication's dissolution in the patient's body.

Common Lubricants:

Magnesium stearate: The most widely used pharmaceutical lubricant, magnesium stearate is a salt derived from stearic acid (often obtained from animal sources). While generally well-tolerated, some patients experience allergic reactions, and there are concerns about its potential to interfere with medication absorption when used in massive quantities.

Stearic acid: Used alone or in combination with magnesium stearate, stearic acid can cause digestive upset in sensitive individuals and may affect the dissolution rate of medications.

Talc: A mineral lubricant that has largely been phased out of pharmaceutical use due to concerns about contamination with asbestos and respiratory risks but still appears in some older formulations and overseas-manufactured medications.

Sodium stearyl fumarate: A newer lubricant designed to address some of the concerns with magnesium stearate, but with limited long-term safety data for pharmaceutical applications.

Coatings: The Outer Shell

Many modern medications feature sophisticated coating systems that serve multiple purposes: protecting the active ingredient from moisture and light, controlling dissolution timing, masking unpleasant tastes, and improving the medication's appearance.

Common Coating Materials:

Hydroxypropyl methylcellulose (HPMC): Used in film coatings that provide moisture protection and improve swallowability. Can cause allergic reactions in sensitive individuals.

Polyethylene glycol (PEG): A polymer used in coating formulations that can cause allergic reactions ranging from skin rashes to severe anaphylaxis in susceptible patients.

Titanium dioxide: A white pigment used to provide opacity and color to medication coatings. While approved for pharmaceutical use, titanium dioxide has been classified as a possible carcinogen by some international health agencies.

Iron oxides: Mineral pigments used to provide assorted colors to medication coatings. These can cause allergic reactions in patients sensitive to iron compounds.

Shellac: A natural resin used in enteric coatings designed to protect medications from stomach acid. Shellac can cause allergic reactions and is problematic for patients with shellfish allergies who may cross-react with this substance.

The Allergen Minefield

For patients with food allergies, sensitivities, or dietary restrictions, medications represent a hidden minefield of problematic substances that are rarely disclosed in plain language. The technical names used for pharmaceutical ingredients often obscure their origins, making it nearly impossible for patients and even healthcare providers to identify potential allergens.

Lactose: The Hidden Dairy

Lactose appears in an estimated 70% of prescription medications and 20% of over-the-counter drugs. For the approximately 65% of adults worldwide who experience some degree of lactose intolerance, this hidden dairy consumption can cause significant digestive symptoms that are often misattributed to medication side effects or underlying health conditions.

The amount of lactose in medications can be substantial. Some tablets contain 100-200 milligrams of lactose each, meaning patients taking multiple medications might consume several grams of lactose daily equivalent to drinking a small glass of milk.

Gluten: The Grain Connection

Gluten-containing ingredients appear in many medications through wheat-derived starches, binding agents, and coating materials. For patients with celiac disease or non-celiac gluten sensitivity, consuming these medications can trigger immune reactions that cause intestinal damage and systemic symptoms.

The challenge for gluten-sensitive patients is that pharmaceutical labeling rarely identifies the source of starch-based ingredients. An ingredient listed as "starch" could be derived from corn (gluten-free), wheat (contains gluten), or other grains, with no way for patients to determine which without contacting manufacturers directly.

Artificial Dyes: The Petroleum Products

Many medications contain artificial colors derived from petroleum products, including:

FD&C Red No. 40: Linked to hyperactivity in children and allergic reactions in sensitive individuals

FD&C Yellow No. 6: Associated with allergic reactions and behavioral problems

FD&C Blue No. 1: Can cause allergic reactions and has been linked to attention problems in some studies

These dyes serve no medical purpose—they're added purely for cosmetic reasons to make medications more visually appealing or to help distinguish between different strengths or formulations.

Why "Inactive" Doesn't Mean Harmless

The fundamental problem with the inactive ingredient designation is that it confuses therapeutic activity with biological activity. While these substances may not contribute to the medication's intended therapeutic effect, they absolutely interact with your body in measurable ways.

Biological Activities of "Inactive" Ingredients:

Immune system activation: Many pharmaceutical excipients can trigger allergic reactions, autoimmune responses, or inflammatory processes that have nothing to do with the medication's intended purpose.

Digestive system effects: Fillers, binders, and other excipients can affect gut bacteria, intestinal permeability, and digestive function in ways that impact overall health.

Absorption interference: Some inactive ingredients can alter how quickly or completely the active ingredient is absorbed, potentially affecting the medication's effectiveness.

Metabolic interactions: Excipients can interact with liver enzymes, kidney function, and other metabolic processes, potentially affecting how the body processes both the medication and other substances.

Cumulative toxicity: Regular consumption of certain excipients over months or years may lead to accumulation in body tissues with unknown long-term consequences.

Individual Sensitivity: The Personal Equation

One of the most troubling aspects of the inactive ingredient problem is how it affects individual patients differently. Two people can take the same medication and have completely different experiences based on their sensitivity to various excipients, yet this individual variation is rarely considered in prescribing decisions.

Factors That Affect Sensitivity:

Genetic variations: People metabolize chemicals differently based on genetic factors that affect enzyme production, immune system function, and other biological processes.

Existing health conditions: Patients with compromised immune systems, digestive disorders, kidney problems, or liver dysfunction may be more susceptible to adverse effects from pharmaceutical excipients.

Age-related changes: Children and elderly patients often process chemicals differently than healthy adults, potentially making them more vulnerable to excipient-related problems.

Medication load: Patients taking multiple medications are exposed to much higher levels of excipients than those taking single medications, increasing the risk of cumulative effects.

Environmental factors: Exposure to pollution, chemicals, and other environmental toxins can affect how individuals respond to pharmaceutical additives.

Cumulative Exposure: The Mounting Chemical Load

Perhaps the most concerning aspect of pharmaceutical excipient exposure is the cumulative effect of consuming multiple inactive ingredients across different medications over extended periods. While individual excipients might be safe in isolation, no one has studied the safety of consuming dozens of different pharmaceutical chemicals simultaneously over years or decades.

The Daily Chemical Cocktail:

Consider a typical patient taking five common medications:

Morning blood pressure medication: Contains lactose, microcrystalline cellulose, magnesium stearate, and artificial coloring

Diabetes medication: Contains corn starch, povidone, talc, and titanium dioxide

Cholesterol medication: Contains calcium carbonate, hydroxypropyl cellulose, and polyethylene glycol

Pain reliever: Contains sodium starch glycolate, croscarmellose sodium, and iron oxide

Multivitamin: Contains gelatin, glycerin, soybean oil, and various preservatives

This patient is consuming at least 15-20 different pharmaceutical chemicals daily, many in substantial quantities, with no evaluation of how these substances might interact with each other or accumulate in body tissues over time.

The Research Gap

Despite the widespread use of pharmaceutical excipients and growing concerns about their safety, remarkably little research has been conducted on their long-term health effects, particularly in combination with other chemicals or in vulnerable populations.

What We Don't Know:

Long-term effects of daily consumption of pharmaceutical excipients over years or decades

Interaction effects between different excipients consumed simultaneously

Cumulative toxicity of excipients that may accumulate in body tissues

Effects on vulnerable populations including children, elderly, and immunocompromised patients

Impact on gut microbiome and digestive health

Potential for excipients to interfere with the effectiveness of active ingredients

Environmental and occupational health effects of excipient manufacturing

This research gap exists because pharmaceutical companies have no financial incentive to study the safety of excipients beyond basic toxicity testing, and regulatory agencies don't require such studies for approval.

Protecting Yourself

Given the current state of knowledge about pharmaceutical excipients, patients who want to minimize their exposure to potentially problematic inactive ingredients face significant challenges. However, there are steps you can take to reduce your risk:

Know Your Sensitivities: Work with healthcare providers to identify specific ingredients that cause problems for you and maintain a list of substances to avoid.

Read Labels Carefully: Learn to recognize the technical names for common allergens and problematic substances in pharmaceutical ingredients.

Ask Pharmacists: Pharmacists often have access to more detailed ingredient information than what appears on standard labels and can help identify alternatives.

Consider Compounding: Custom-compounded medications can eliminate problematic excipients, though this option may be more expensive and isn't available for all medications.

Monitor Symptoms: Keep track of any unusual symptoms that might be related to inactive ingredients rather than active medication effects.

The Manufacturing Contamination Factor

Beyond the intentionally added excipients lies another layer of chemical complexity that pharmaceutical companies rarely discuss manufacturing contaminants and processing residues that remain in finished medications. These substances aren't listed on labels because they're not supposed to be there, but they're present nonetheless due to the realities of industrial pharmaceutical production.

Solvent Residues

Pharmaceutical manufacturing uses various industrial solvents to extract, purify, and process active ingredients. While these solvents are supposed to be removed during production, complete elimination is often impossible or economically impractical. The FDA allows "acceptable" levels of solvent residues in finished medications, but these limits are based on industrial exposure standards rather than standards appropriate for daily consumption by sick patients.

Common solvent residues found in medications include:

Methanol: A toxic alcohol that can cause blindness and organ damage even in tiny amounts

Acetone: An industrial solvent that can affect the nervous system and respiratory function

Toluene: A petroleum-derived solvent linked to neurological problems and reproductive issues

Ethyl acetate: A solvent that can cause respiratory irritation and nervous system effects

The cumulative exposure to these solvent residues across multiple medications has never been studied, yet patients taking several different medications may consume significant quantities of these industrial chemicals over time.

Heavy Metal Contamination

Pharmaceutical manufacturing processes often involve catalysts and processing aids that contain heavy metals. These substances can leave trace residues in finished medications that accumulate in body tissues over time. Common heavy metal contaminants include:

Lead: Even tiny amounts can affect neurological development and function

Mercury: Particularly dangerous for pregnant women and children

Cadmium: A known carcinogen that accumulates in kidneys and other organs

Arsenic: Present in some medications as a processing contaminant

The pharmaceutical industry argues that these contamination levels are "negligible," but this assessment doesn't consider the cumulative exposure from multiple medications or the increased vulnerability of sick patients whose bodies may be less able to eliminate these toxins.

Bacterial Endotoxins

Manufacturing facilities that don't maintain adequate sterility can introduce bacterial contamination into medications. Even when the bacteria themselves are killed during processing, their toxic breakdown products (endotoxins) can remain in finished medications and cause inflammatory reactions in patients.

These endotoxins are particularly problematic for patients with compromised immune systems, autoimmune conditions, or chronic inflammatory diseases. What appears to be a side effect of the active ingredient may actually be an inflammatory response to bacterial contaminants in the medication.

The Dosage Form Deception

The way medications are formulated and delivered to patients creates additional opportunities for chemical exposure that most people never consider. Each dosage form—tablets, capsules, liquids, patches—requires its own set of specialized chemicals to function properly.

Capsule Chemistry

Gelatin capsules, while appearing simple, contain numerous chemical additives:

Gelatin: Usually derived from animal sources, potentially exposing patients to prion diseases, animal hormones, and other biological contaminants

Plasticizers: Chemical softening agents that keep gelatin flexible but may have hormone-disrupting effects

Preservatives: Anti-microbial agents that prevent bacterial growth in the gelatin

Opacifiers: Substances that make capsules opaque, often including titanium dioxide

Colorants: Artificial dyes that serve no medical purpose but may cause allergic reactions

Vegetarian capsules made from plant cellulose aren't necessarily safer—they often contain chemical cross-linking agents, stabilizers, and other processing aids that may be poorly tolerated by sensitive individuals.

Liquid Medication Complexity

Liquid medications present unique formulation challenges that require extensive use of chemical additives:

Preservatives: Liquid formulations are particularly susceptible to bacterial and fungal contamination, requiring powerful antimicrobial agents

Stabilizers: Many active ingredients are unstable in liquid form, requiring chemical stabilizers to prevent degradation

Solubilizers: Substances that help dissolve ingredients that would otherwise separate or precipitate

Viscosity modifiers: Chemicals that control the thickness and flow properties of liquid medications

pH adjusters: Acids and bases used to maintain proper acidity levels for stability and absorption

Children's liquid medications are often the worst offenders, containing elevated levels of artificial sweeteners, dyes, and preservatives to make them palatable and visually appealing to young patients.

Transdermal Patch Technology

Medication patches that deliver drugs through the skin require sophisticated chemical systems:

Penetration enhancers: Chemicals that disrupt skin barriers to allow drug absorption

Adhesives: Often contain allergenic substances that can cause contact dermatitis

Backing materials: Synthetic polymers that may contain plasticizers and other additives

Rate-controlling membranes: Synthetic materials that regulate drug release but may contain industrial chemicals

The Generic Medication Wild Card

Generic medications present unique challenges for patients trying to avoid problematic inactive ingredients. While generic drugs must contain the same active ingredient as brand-name medications, they can use completely different excipients, potentially exposing patients to new allergens and chemical sensitivities.

The Substitution Problem

When pharmacies substitute generic medications for brand-name drugs, patients often receive medications with entirely different inactive ingredient profiles. Someone who has successfully taken a brand-name medication for years might suddenly experience new symptoms when switched to a generic version that contains different fillers, binders, or preservatives.

This substitution can occur without patient knowledge or consent, and healthcare providers are rarely informed about the specific inactive ingredients in the generic medications they prescribe. The result is a system where patients can unknowingly be exposed to new chemical sensitivities every time they fill a prescription.

Manufacturing Variability

Different generic manufacturers may use completely different excipient systems for the same medication. Two generic versions of the same drug might contain entirely different sets of inactive ingredients, making it impossible for patients to predict their response to a new generic formulation.

This variability is particularly problematic for patients with multiple chemical sensitivities who have learned to avoid specific excipients. They may successfully identify and avoid problematic ingredients in one generic formulation, only to be exposed to different problematic substances when their pharmacy switches to a different generic manufacturer.

The Pediatric Chemical Burden

Children face unique risks from pharmaceutical excipients because their developing bodies process chemicals differently than adults, yet most excipient safety data is based on adult exposure patterns. Children's medications often contain higher levels of sweeteners, dyes, and preservatives to improve palatability, potentially exposing developing nervous systems to chemicals that may affect behavior and cognitive function.

Weight-Based Exposure Differences

Children receive much higher dose-per-kilogram exposure to pharmaceutical excipients than adults. A 30-pound child taking the same tablet as a 150-pound adult receives five times the excipient exposure relative to body weight. This dramatically increased exposure occurs during critical developmental periods when children's brains and organs are most vulnerable to chemical interference.

Behavioral and Cognitive Effects

Growing evidence suggests that artificial dyes, preservatives, and other pharmaceutical additives may contribute to attention problems, hyperactivity, and learning difficulties in susceptible children. Yet these substances continue to be used routinely in pediatric medications because they improve compliance and reduce manufacturing costs.

The irony is striking children being treated for attention deficit disorders may be consuming medications that contain chemicals known to worsen attention and behavioral problems in sensitive individuals.

The Elderly Vulnerability Factor

Elderly patients face increased risks from pharmaceutical excipients due to age-related changes in metabolism, kidney function, and immune system response. As people age, their ability to eliminate chemicals from their bodies decreases, potentially leading to accumulation of excipients that would be safely processed by younger patients.

Polypharmacy Amplification

Elderly patients often take multiple medications simultaneously, dramatically increasing their exposure to pharmaceutical excipients. Someone taking ten different medications might consume dozens of different chemical additives daily, creating exposure levels that have never been tested for safety in any population.

The combination of decreased chemical elimination capacity and increased chemical exposure creates a perfect storm for excipient-related health problems in elderly patients. Symptoms that might be attributed to aging or disease progression could actually result from cumulative chemical toxicity.

The Autoimmune Connection

Emerging research suggests that repeated exposure to pharmaceutical excipients may contribute to the development of autoimmune conditions in susceptible individuals. Many excipients act as adjuvants—substances that stimulate immune system activity—and chronic exposure to these immune stimulants may trigger autoimmune responses in genetically predisposed patients.

This connection is particularly concerning given the rising rates of autoimmune diseases in developed countries and the concurrent increase in pharmaceutical consumption. While correlation doesn't prove causation, the potential for pharmaceutical excipients to contribute to autoimmune disease development deserves serious investigation that isn't currently being conducted.

Environmental and Occupational Exposures

The chemicals used as pharmaceutical excipients don't disappear when patients consume medications—they're excreted in urine and feces, entering wastewater systems and potentially affecting environmental and drinking water quality. Workers in pharmaceutical manufacturing facilities face occupational exposure to these chemicals at much higher levels than patients, yet occupational safety data is rarely considered when evaluating the safety of pharmaceutical excipients for consumer use.

Breaking the Cycle

The inactive ingredient myth persists because it serves the interests of pharmaceutical companies, regulatory agencies, and healthcare providers who prefer simple explanations over complex chemical realities. Breaking this cycle requires fundamental changes in how we think about pharmaceutical safety:

Transparency Requirements: Pharmaceutical companies should be required to disclose all ingredients in plain language, including their sources and potential allergens.

Individual Risk Assessment: Healthcare providers should routinely assess patients' sensitivity to pharmaceutical excipients before prescribing medications.

Alternative Formulations: More medications should be available in multiple formulations to accommodate patients with specific chemical sensitivities.

Long-term Safety Studies: Independent research should evaluate the long-term effects of consuming pharmaceutical excipients, particularly in combination and in vulnerable populations.

The inactive ingredient myth represents one of the most pervasive and dangerous misconceptions in modern medicine. These substances are far from inactive—they're biologically active compounds that can significantly impact your health, particularly when consumed regularly over extended periods. Until the medical system acknowledges this reality and begins treating pharmaceutical excipients with the caution they deserve, patients must advocate for themselves and make informed decisions about the chemical risks they're willing to accept along with their medications.

Chapter 5: Colors, Flavors, and Preservatives

When I first started examining my medications closely, one thing struck me immediately: they looked nothing like medicine should look. My blood pressure pills were bright blue. My anti-inflammatory was hot pink. My vitamins came in an array of colors that would make a rainbow jealous. These weren't the plain white tablets I remembered from childhood—they were colorful, artificially flavored, and designed to be visually appealing.

It dawned on me that pharmaceutical companies were spending enormous amounts of money making their products look and taste like candy. But unlike candy, which you might eat occasionally as a treat, these were substances I was supposed to consume daily for months or years. The chemicals responsible for those appealing colors, pleasant flavors, and extended shelf lives weren't there for my health—they were there for marketing, manufacturing convenience, and corporate profits.

What I discovered about the dyes, artificial flavors, and preservatives in medications shocked me more than the hidden soy and dairy. These substances serve no medical purpose whatsoever. They exist solely to make medications more marketable and profitable, yet they carry real health risks that patients are never warned about. Worse, many of these cosmetic chemicals have been banned in food products in other countries due to safety concerns, yet they remain perfectly legal in American medications.

The Psychology of Pharmaceutical Aesthetics

The pharmaceutical industry has borrowed heavily from food and cosmetics marketing, recognizing that patients' willingness to take medications is significantly influenced by their appearance, taste, and smell. This has led to an entire sub-industry focused on making medications as appealing as possible rather than as safe as possible.

Color Psychology in Medicine

Pharmaceutical companies employ teams of psychologists and marketing experts to determine the optimal colors for their medications. Research shows that patients associate distinct colors with different effects: red pills are perceived as stimulating, blue pills as calming, and white pills as weak or ineffective. These associations have nothing to do with the actual chemical properties of the medications, but they significantly influence patient compliance and satisfaction.

The result is a medication landscape where colors are chosen based on marketing research rather than medical necessity. A blood pressure medication might be colored blue to suggest calmness and cardiovascular health, even though the blue dye serves no therapeutic purpose and may actually cause health problems in sensitive patients.

The Compliance Deception

Pharmaceutical companies justify the use of artificial colors and flavors by claiming they improve "patient compliance"—the likelihood that patients will take their medications as prescribed. The logic is that medications that look and taste appealing are more likely to be taken regularly, leading to better health outcomes.

This argument conveniently ignores several important considerations: First, it treats patients like children who can't make rational decisions about their health based on medical necessity rather than candy-like appeal. Second, it prioritizes short-term compliance over long-term safety, potentially exposing patients to unnecessary chemical risks. Third, it assumes that making medications appealing is worth the health risks associated with artificial additives.

Artificial Dyes: Petroleum in Your Pills

The bright colors that make modern medications so visually appealing come primarily from artificial dyes derived from petroleum products. These synthetic colorants have been linked to a wide range of health problems, yet they continue to be used extensively in pharmaceuticals because they're cheap, stable, and effective at creating appealing appearances.

The Major Culprits

FD&C Red No. 40 (Allura Red AC): The most widely used artificial dye in American medications, Red 40 is derived from petroleum and coal tar. Studies have linked this dye to hyperactivity in children, allergic reactions, and possible carcinogenic effects. It's been banned in several European countries for use in children's products, yet it remains common in American pediatric medications.

FD&C Yellow No. 6 (Sunset Yellow FCF): Another petroleum-derived dye that has been associated with hyperactivity, attention problems, and allergic reactions. Some studies suggest it may also affect reproductive health and cause chromosomal damage. Like Red 40, it's restricted or banned in many European countries but widely used in American medications.

FD&C Blue No. 1 (Brilliant Blue FCF): Used to create the appealing blue color in many medications, this dye has been linked to allergic reactions and may affect the nervous system. Studies in animals have shown it can cross the blood-brain barrier, raising concerns about its effects on brain function.

FD&C Yellow No. 5 (Tartrazine): Perhaps the most notorious artificial dye, Yellow 5 is known to cause severe allergic reactions in sensitive individuals, including hives, asthma attacks, and behavioral problems. It's been linked to attention deficit disorders and hyperactivity in children.

FD&C Green No. 3 (Fast Green FCF): Less commonly used but equally problematic, this dye has been associated with bladder tumors in animal studies and allergic reactions in humans.

The Hidden Health Costs

The health implications of consuming artificial dyes daily through medications are far more serious than most patients realize. Unlike occasional exposure through colored foods, medication use involves regular, long-term consumption of these chemicals, often in higher concentrations than found in food products.

Neurological Effects: Multiple studies have demonstrated links between artificial food dyes and attention problems, hyperactivity, and learning difficulties in children. The mechanism appears to involve disruption of neurotransmitter function and increased brain inflammation. For children taking colored medications daily, this exposure may exacerbate the very conditions their medications are supposed to treat.

Allergic Reactions: Artificial dyes are among the most common causes of food and drug allergies. Reactions can range from mild skin rashes to severe anaphylaxis. Many patients who experience "drug allergies" may actually be reacting to the artificial colors rather than the active ingredients.

Carcinogenic Potential: Several artificial dyes have shown carcinogenic effects in animal studies. While the cancer risk from medication dyes hasn't been specifically studied in humans, the regular consumption of potentially carcinogenic substances through daily medications represents an unnecessary and preventable risk.

Immune System Disruption: Artificial dyes can act as immune system stimulants, potentially triggering autoimmune reactions and chronic inflammation. For patients with existing autoimmune conditions, this additional immune stimulation may worsen their underlying disease.

Preservatives: Trading Shelf Life for Health

Medications, particularly liquid formulations, require preservatives to prevent bacterial and fungal growth during storage and use. While some preservation is necessary for safety, the pharmaceutical industry often uses preservatives that extend shelf life far beyond what's medically necessary, prioritizing product economics over patient health.

The Preservative Arsenal

Parabens (Methylparaben, Propylparaben, Butylparaben): These widely used preservatives have been shown to mimic estrogen in the body, potentially disrupting hormonal balance and contributing to reproductive health problems. Parabens have been found in breast cancer tissue, though a direct causal link hasn't been definitively established. Several European countries have banned or restricted parabens in consumer products, yet they remain common in American medications.

Benzyl Alcohol: Used as both a preservative and solvent, benzyl alcohol can cause serious neurological problems, particularly in infants and children. It has been linked to "gasping syndrome" in premature babies and can cause CNS depression and metabolic acidosis. Despite these risks, it's commonly used in pediatric medications.

Formaldehyde-Releasing Preservatives: Several preservatives work by slowly releasing formaldehyde, a known carcinogen. These include:

DMDM hydantoin

Diazolidinyl urea

Imidazolidinyl urea

Quaternium-15

The continuous release of formaldehyde from these preservatives means patients are exposed to this carcinogen every time they take their medication. The cumulative exposure from multiple medications containing these preservatives has never been studied.

Sodium Benzoate: When combined with vitamin C (ascorbic acid), sodium benzoate can form benzene, a known carcinogen. Many medications contain both substances, creating the potential for benzene formation under certain storage conditions. This combination is restricted in European pharmaceuticals but remains common in American products.

Thimerosal: A mercury-containing preservative that was largely removed from vaccines due to safety concerns but continues to be used in some medications and eye drops. Mercury is a potent neurotoxin that can accumulate in body tissues, yet some patients continue to be exposed through their daily medications.

The Preservation Paradox

The most troubling aspect of pharmaceutical preservatives is that many are used at concentrations far higher than necessary for basic preservation. Pharmaceutical companies choose preservative systems based on manufacturing convenience and shelf-life extension rather than minimum effective concentrations for patient safety.

This approach means patients are exposed to unnecessarily high levels of potentially harmful preservatives simply because manufacturers want to extend product shelf life for economic reasons. A medication that could be safely preserved with lower concentrations of less toxic preservatives instead contains high levels of more dangerous substances because they're cheaper or provide longer shelf stability.

Sweeteners and Flavoring: The Artificial Taste Revolution

Liquid medications, particularly those designed for children, contain extensive artificial flavoring and sweetening systems designed to mask the bitter or unpleasant taste of active ingredients. These flavoring systems often represent a sizable portion of the medication's volume and expose patients to a complex mixture of synthetic chemicals.

Artificial Sweeteners

Aspartame: One of the most controversial artificial sweeteners, aspartame has been linked to headaches, seizures, mood disorders, and neurological problems. It breaks down into methanol and formaldehyde in the body, both toxic substances. Despite safety concerns, it's widely used in sugar-free liquid medications and chewable tablets.

Sucralose: Marketed as a safer alternative to aspartame, sucralose is a chlorinated sugar compound that has been associated with digestive problems, immune system disruption, and potential effects on gut bacteria. Some studies suggest it may interfere with glucose metabolism, which could be particularly problematic for diabetic patients taking sucralose-containing medications.

Acesulfame Potassium (Ace-K): This artificial sweetener contains methylene chloride, a potential carcinogen. Studies have suggested links to cancer, mood disorders, and liver problems. It's often used in combination with other artificial sweeteners to create more palatable flavoring systems.

Saccharin: The oldest artificial sweetener, saccharin has been linked to bladder cancer in animal studies. While it remains approved for human use, many countries have restrictions on its use in consumer products.

Artificial Flavoring Systems

The "natural and artificial flavors" listed on medication labels often represent complex mixtures of dozens or even hundreds of individual chemical compounds. These flavoring systems are considered trade secrets, so patients and healthcare providers have no way to know exactly what chemicals they contain.

Common Artificial Flavoring Chemicals:

Vanillin: Synthetic vanilla flavoring that can cause allergic reactions and may interfere with liver function when consumed regularly in significant quantities.

Ethyl Butyrate: Creates fruity flavors but can cause respiratory irritation and nervous system effects.

Benzaldehyde: Provides almond and cherry flavoring but can cause CNS depression and respiratory problems.

Diacetyl: Creates butter and creamy flavors but has been linked to serious lung disease (bronchiolitis obliterans) in workers exposed to it occupationally.

Cinnamaldehyde: Provides cinnamon flavoring but can cause severe allergic reactions and mouth irritation.

The combination of multiple artificial flavoring chemicals creates exposure patterns that have never been studied for safety. Patients taking flavored liquid medications may consume dozens of different synthetic flavoring compounds daily without any evaluation of their cumulative health effects.

Children's Medications: A Special Concern

Perhaps nowhere is the use of unnecessary cosmetic chemicals more troubling than in pediatric medications. Children's formulations are often loaded with artificial colors, flavors, and sweeteners designed to make medicine-taking a pleasant experience rather than a medical necessity.

The Pediatric Chemical Burden

Children face unique vulnerabilities to pharmaceutical additives because their developing nervous systems are more susceptible to chemical interference, their smaller body size means higher dose-per-kilogram exposure, and their immature detoxification systems are less able to eliminate these substances safely.

Behavioral and Cognitive Effects

The connection between artificial dyes and behavioral problems in children has been well-documented in scientific literature. The European Food Safety Authority has concluded that certain artificial dyes can cause hyperactivity and attention problems in children, leading to warning labels on foods containing these substances.

Yet these same dyes continue to be used extensively in American children's medications, often in higher concentrations than found in foods. Children being treated for ADHD may be consuming medications that contain chemicals known to worsen attention and hyperactivity problems.

The Irony of Pediatric Psychopharmacology

Perhaps the most troubling example is the use of artificial dyes in medications prescribed to treat attention and behavioral disorders in children. Many ADHD medications contain Red 40, Yellow 6, and other dyes that have been specifically linked to the symptoms these medications are supposed to treat.

This creates a perverse situation where children may be experiencing medication-induced worsening of their symptoms, leading to higher doses or additional medications to control problems that are actually being caused by unnecessary cosmetic additives in their original prescriptions.

Marketing to Children

Pharmaceutical companies have adopted many of the same marketing techniques used by candy and junk food manufacturers to make children's medications appealing. Bright colors, sweet flavors, and appealing packaging are designed to make children want to take their medications.

While this may improve short-term compliance, it also teaches children to associate medicine with candy-like treats, potentially leading to accidental overdoses when children seek out medications they perceive as treats rather than medicines.

The International Double Standard

The use of artificial colors, flavors, and preservatives in medications varies dramatically between countries, revealing the arbitrary nature of many American safety standards. Substances that are banned or heavily restricted in European medications continue to be used routinely in American products.

European Restrictions

The European Union has implemented much stricter standards for cosmetic additives in medications:

Many artificial dyes require warning labels when used in foods and are banned entirely in medications for children under certain ages

Preservatives like parabens are banned or heavily restricted in pharmaceutical formulations

Artificial sweeteners have stricter usage limits and require specific safety documentation

The Regulatory Arbitrage

Pharmaceutical companies often reformulate their products when selling in countries with stricter standards, proving that these cosmetic additives are unnecessary for the medications' effectiveness. The same company might sell a dye-free, preservative-free version of a medication in Europe while continuing to use artificial additives in the American version.

This regulatory arbitrage demonstrates that the use of these chemicals is driven by economic and marketing considerations rather than medical necessity. If a medication can be safely and effectively produced without artificial dyes and preservatives for European markets, there's no medical reason to include these substances in American formulations.

The Economics of Aesthetics

The pharmaceutical industry's investment in cosmetic additives reveals important priorities about profit versus patient safety. Companies spend millions of dollars researching optimal colors, flavors, and preservative systems while conducting minimal research on the long-term health effects of these substances.

Marketing Budget Allocation

Pharmaceutical companies often spend more money on the cosmetic aspects of their medications than on safety testing of these additives. Focus groups, color psychology research, and flavor optimization studies receive substantial funding, while long-term safety studies of artificial additives are largely neglected.

The Compliance Myth

While pharmaceutical companies justify cosmetic additives by claiming they improve patient compliance, independent research suggests that patient education and support programs are far more effective at improving medication adherence than making pills look and taste appealing.

The emphasis on cosmetic appeal represents a fundamental misunderstanding of patient motivation. Most patients take medications because they understand the health benefits, not because the pills are pretty or taste good. For patients who are non-compliant due to side effects or lack of efficacy, artificial colors and flavors do nothing to address the underlying problems.

Protecting Yourself and Your Family

Given the current regulatory environment that allows extensive use of unnecessary cosmetic chemicals in medications, patients who want to minimize their exposure face significant challenges. However, there are strategies you can employ:

Request Dye-Free Formulations: Many medications are available in both colored and dye-free versions. Ask your pharmacist about alternatives that don't contain artificial colors.

Read Labels Carefully: Learn to identify artificial dyes, preservatives, and flavoring agents on medication labels. Common names to watch for include FD&C colors, parabens, artificial flavors, and formaldehyde-releasing preservatives.

Consider Compounding: Custom-compounded medications can eliminate unnecessary additives while maintaining therapeutic effectiveness. This option may be more expensive but can be essential for patients with multiple chemical sensitivities.

Advocate for Children: Be particularly vigilant about cosmetic additives in children's medications. Request dye-free, sugar-free formulations whenever possible, and question whether flavored liquid medications are necessary.

Document Reactions: Keep track of any symptoms that might be related to medication additives rather than active ingredients. This information can help guide future medication choices and may reveal patterns that healthcare providers miss.

Support Regulatory Reform: Contact legislators and regulatory agencies to advocate for stricter standards regarding cosmetic additives in medications, particularly for children's formulations.

The Manufacturing Conspiracy

The extensive use of cosmetic chemicals in medications isn't accidental—it's the result of deliberate decisions by pharmaceutical companies to prioritize appearance and marketability over patient safety. Internal company documents obtained through litigation have revealed the calculated nature of these choices and the industry's awareness of potential health risks.

Marketing Over Medicine

Pharmaceutical companies employ teams of marketing specialists, color psychologists, and flavor chemists whose job is to make medications as appealing as possible. These professionals work closely with manufacturing teams to develop formulations that maximize visual and sensory appeal, often with little input from medical or safety experts.

Meeting minutes from major pharmaceutical companies show discussions about color selection that focus entirely on market research and consumer preferences, with no mention of health implications. Companies routinely choose more appealing but potentially more dangerous additives over safer alternatives when market testing shows improved patient acceptance.

The Flavor Industry Connection

The artificial flavoring systems used in medications come from the same companies that create flavors for junk food, candy, and processed foods. These flavor houses specialize in creating addictive taste profiles designed to encourage repeated consumption—exactly the opposite of what should guide medication development.

Many pharmaceutical flavoring agents are borrowed directly from the food industry without any modification for medical use. A strawberry flavoring system originally designed to make children crave more candy is used unchanged in pediatric antibiotics, creating medications that children may seek out for their taste rather than their medical necessity.

The Hidden Addiction Factor

What pharmaceutical companies don't advertise is that many of the artificial flavoring and sweetening agents used in medications can create psychological and physiological dependencies that have nothing to do with the therapeutic effects of the drugs themselves.

Artificial Sweetener Dependencies

Artificial sweeteners like aspartame and sucralose can alter brain chemistry in ways that create cravings for sweet tastes. Patients taking sweetened liquid medications may develop dependencies on the sweetening agents that make them resistant to switching to unsweetened alternatives.

This artificial sweetener dependency can be particularly problematic for diabetic patients who are trying to reduce their overall sugar and artificial sweetener consumption. Their diabetes medications may be working against their dietary goals by maintaining cravings for artificial sweetness.

Flavor Conditioning

The psychological conditioning created by pleasant-tasting medications can interfere with patients' ability to make rational decisions about their treatment. When medications taste good, patients may be more likely to continue taking them even when they're experiencing side effects or when the medications are no longer medically necessary.

Conversely, when patients become accustomed to sweet, flavored medications, they may resist taking necessary medications that don't have appealing tastes, even when those medications might be safer or more effective.

The Regulatory Capture Problem

The continued use of dangerous cosmetic chemicals in medications is facilitated by regulatory capture—the process by which industries gain influence over the agencies supposed to regulate them. The pharmaceutical industry's influence over the FDA extends to cosmetic additive approval and safety standards.

Industry-Funded Safety Studies

Most of the safety data on pharmaceutical cosmetic additives comes from studies funded by the companies that profit from their use. These studies typically focus on acute toxicity—whether substances cause immediate harm in large doses—rather than the chronic health effects of daily consumption over years or decades.

Independent researchers who attempt to study the long-term effects of pharmaceutical additives often find themselves blocked by industry claims of trade secrets and proprietary information. This creates a system where safety assessments are controlled by the companies with the greatest financial interest in positive outcomes.

The Revolving Door Effect

Many FDA officials responsible for approving cosmetic additives in medications later take jobs with pharmaceutical companies or consulting firms that serve the industry. This revolving door creates conflicts of interest that influence regulatory decisions in favor of industry preferences rather than patient safety.

Former FDA officials often use their regulatory expertise to help pharmaceutical companies navigate approval processes for new cosmetic additives or to challenge proposed restrictions on existing substances. This system ensures that industry interests are well-represented in regulatory discussions while patient safety advocates have little influence.

The International Shame

The contrast between American and international standards for pharmaceutical cosmetic additives represents a national embarrassment that reveals how thoroughly the pharmaceutical industry has captured American regulatory processes.

The European Model

European pharmaceutical regulations require companies to justify the necessity of every cosmetic additive and demonstrate that safer alternatives aren't available. This approach has led to the development of numerous additive-free formulations that are just as effective as their American counterparts.

European patients can access dye-free, preservative-free, and artificially-sweetener-free versions of most common medications, proving that these additives are unnecessary for therapeutic effectiveness. The same pharmaceutical companies that claim cosmetic additives are essential for American patients somehow manage to produce effective medications without them for European markets.

The Canadian Contrast

Even Canada, with a regulatory system similar to the United States, has implemented stricter standards for pharmaceutical cosmetic additives. Canadian regulations require clearer labeling of artificial additives and mandate safer alternatives when they're available.

The proximity of Canadian and American markets means that pharmaceutical companies often produce the same medications with different additive profiles for each country. American patients are essentially being used as test subjects for cosmetic additives that are considered too dangerous for use in neighboring countries.

The Path Forward

The current system that allows extensive use of unnecessary cosmetic chemicals in medications represents a triumph of marketing over medicine. These substances serve no therapeutic purpose while exposing patients to avoidable health risks, yet they remain ubiquitous in American pharmaceuticals because they increase profits and improve marketability.

Real reform will require fundamental changes in how we prioritize pharmaceutical safety over cosmetic appeal. Medications should be judged by their therapeutic effectiveness and safety profile, not by their visual appeal or taste. Until we recognize that medicine isn't candy and doesn't need to look or taste like candy, patients will continue to be exposed to unnecessary chemical risks in pursuit of pharmaceutical industry profits.

Immediate Action Steps

Patients can begin protecting themselves immediately by demanding additive-free formulations, supporting regulatory reform efforts, and educating healthcare providers about the risks of cosmetic pharmaceutical chemicals. Healthcare systems can implement policies that prioritize additive-free medications and require justification for any cosmetic additives used in patient care.

Regulatory agencies must be forced to acknowledge that cosmetic appeal is not a valid reason to expose patients to potential health risks. Safety standards should be based on the most protective international models rather than the most permissive industry preferences.

The next time you pick up a colorful, sweet-tasting medication, remember that those appealing characteristics come from petroleum-derived dyes, synthetic flavoring chemicals, and preservatives that may be more dangerous than the condition you're trying to treat. In a rational healthcare system, medications would be as simple as possible, containing only what's necessary for therapeutic effect. Instead, we have a system that prioritizes marketing appeal over patient safety, turning essential medicines into chemical cocktails designed to maximize profits rather than minimize risks.

Chapter 6: Manufacturing Contaminants

During my years of taking various medications after my 18 surgeries, I always assumed that if something was wrong with my pills, I'd know it immediately. I imagined contamination as something obvious—discolored tablets, strange smells, or visible foreign particles. What I never considered was that the most dangerous contamination would be completely invisible, odorless, and tasteless, silently exposing me and millions of other patients to cancer-causing chemicals that had no business being in our medications.

The reality of pharmaceutical contamination is far more insidious than most patients realize. We're not talking about obvious manufacturing errors that get caught by quality control systems. We're talking about systematic contamination that can persist for years, affecting millions of patients before anyone notices there's a problem. These contaminants aren't accidents—they're the predictable result of manufacturing processes that prioritize cost and speed over purity and safety.

What makes this contamination crisis particularly outrageous is that pharmaceutical companies often know about contamination problems long before they inform regulators or patients. Internal company documents obtained through litigation have revealed instances where manufacturers discovered dangerous contaminants in their products but continued shipping them to patients while conducting their own "risk assessments" to determine whether the contamination was "commercially viable" to address.

The NDMA Crisis: Cancer in Every Pill

In 2018, the pharmaceutical world was rocked by the discovery that millions of patients had been consuming probable carcinogens in their daily blood pressure medications. N-Nitrosodimethylamine (NDMA), a chemical so dangerous that it's used to induce cancer in laboratory animals, was found in massive quantities in generic versions of popular blood pressure medications.

What made this discovery particularly shocking wasn't just the presence of NDMA—it was the amounts involved and the duration of exposure. Some batches of contaminated medications contained NDMA levels thousands of times higher than what's considered acceptable for daily consumption. Patients who had been taking these medications as prescribed for years had unknowingly consumed enough probable carcinogens to significantly increase their cancer risk.

The Chemical Reality of NDMA

NDMA is classified as a probable human carcinogen by the International Agency for Research on Cancer. It's so reliably cancer-causing that researchers use it specifically to trigger tumor formation in laboratory studies. The compound damages DNA directly and can cause tumors in virtually every organ system, including the liver, kidneys, lungs, and digestive tract.

What makes NDMA particularly dangerous is its potency—even tiny amounts can cause genetic damage that leads to cancer years or decades later. The FDA's "acceptable" daily intake level for NDMA is 96 nanograms per day, roughly equivalent to a few grains of salt. Some contaminated blood pressure medications contained over 17,000 nanograms of NDMA per pill, meaning patients taking these medications as prescribed were consuming nearly 200 times the "safe" limit daily.

How NDMA Gets into Medications

NDMA contamination in pharmaceuticals isn't accidental—it's the predictable result of specific manufacturing processes and chemical reactions. The contamination typically occurs when manufacturers use certain solvents, recycled materials, or specific chemical synthesis pathways that can create NDMA as a byproduct.

In many cases, pharmaceutical companies switched to cheaper manufacturing processes that were known to create higher risks of NDMA formation. These process changes were motivated by cost reduction rather than safety improvement, and companies often failed to adequately test for NDMA formation when implementing new manufacturing methods.

The most troubling aspect of NDMA contamination is that it often occurs in facilities that have passed FDA inspections. NDMA isn't something that standard quality control testing typically looks for, so contaminated medications can pass all routine safety checks while still containing dangerous levels of carcinogens.

The Broader Nitrosamine Problem

NDMA was just the beginning. As regulators began testing more systematically for nitrosamine contamination, they discovered a widespread problem affecting dozens of different medications. N-Nitrosodiethylamine (NDEA), N-Nitrosodiisopropylamine (NDIPA), and other nitrosamine compounds were found in blood pressure medications, diabetes drugs, heartburn medications, and other common prescriptions.

The Ranitidine Disaster

Perhaps the most devastating nitrosamine contamination involved ranitidine, the active ingredient in the popular heartburn medication Zantac. In 2019, researchers discovered that ranitidine inherently unstable and breaks down to form NDMA, particularly when exposed to heat or stored for extended periods.

This discovery was catastrophic because it meant that ranitidine didn't just contain NDMA as a manufacturing contaminant—the medication itself was a source of NDMA formation. Every patient who had ever taken ranitidine had potentially been exposed to a probable carcinogen, with exposure levels increasing based on storage conditions and medication age.

The ranitidine crisis ultimately led to the complete removal of all ranitidine products from the American market, affecting millions of patients who had been taking these medications for years or decades. But the damage was already done—patients had been consuming NDMA-forming medications for over 30 years before the problem was discovered and addressed.

Metformin Contamination

The diabetes medication metformin presented another troubling example of widespread nitrosamine contamination. Extended-release formulations of metformin from multiple manufacturers were found to contain excessive levels of NDMA, affecting millions of diabetic patients who relied on these medications for blood sugar control.

The metformin contamination was particularly problematic because diabetic patients often take these medications for years or decades, leading to cumulative exposure to carcinogenic compounds over extended periods. Many patients had to switch to different formulations or medications entirely, disrupting established treatment regimens and potentially affecting their diabetes management.

Heavy Metal Contamination: Industrial Toxins in Medicine

While nitrosamine contamination has received significant media attention, heavy metal contamination in medications represents an equally serious but less publicized threat to patient safety. Lead, mercury, cadmium, arsenic, and other toxic metals regularly appear in pharmaceutical products, particularly generic medications manufactured in countries with less stringent environmental and safety controls.

Lead Contamination

Lead contamination in medications is particularly concerning because there is no safe level of lead exposure, especially for children and pregnant women. Even tiny amounts of lead can cause permanent neurological damage, learning disabilities, and behavioral problems.

Multiple recalls of generic medications have been triggered by excessive lead contamination, including popular pain relievers, vitamins, and herbal supplements. In many cases, the lead contamination stems from raw materials sourced from suppliers in countries where environmental lead exposure is widespread due to industrial pollution.

Mercury Poisoning Through Medication

Mercury contamination in pharmaceuticals occurs through several pathways, including the use of mercury-containing preservatives, contaminated raw materials, and industrial processes that use mercury-containing equipment or catalysts.

Some eye drops and nasal sprays still contain thimerosal, a mercury-containing preservative, exposing patients to this potent neurotoxin with every dose. While thimerosal has been largely removed from vaccines due to safety concerns, it continues to be used in other pharmaceutical products with minimal oversight or patient awareness.

Arsenic and Cadmium Exposure

Arsenic and cadmium contamination typically occurs through contaminated raw materials or manufacturing processes that use these elements as catalysts or processing aids. Both metals are known carcinogens that accumulate in body tissues over time, potentially causing cancer and organ damage years after exposure.

The cumulative nature of heavy metal toxicity makes pharmaceutical contamination particularly dangerous. Patients taking multiple contaminated medications over extended periods may develop tissue levels of toxic metals that cause health problems that are never connected to their medication use.

Solvent Residues: Industrial Chemicals in Every Dose

Pharmaceutical manufacturing relies heavily on industrial solvents to extract, purify, and process active ingredients. While these solvents are supposed to be removed during production, complete elimination is often impossible or economically impractical, leaving residual amounts in finished medications.

Common Solvent Contaminants

Methanol: This toxic alcohol can cause blindness, brain damage, and death even in relatively lesser amounts. Methanol residues in medications pose particular risks for patients who consume alcohol or have liver problems that affect their ability to metabolize toxic substances.

Benzene: A known human carcinogen, benzene contamination in medications has triggered multiple recalls. The chemical is particularly dangerous because it can cause leukemia and other blood cancers with relatively low-level chronic exposure.

Toluene: This petroleum-derived solvent can affect the nervous system, causing problems with coordination, cognitive function, and respiratory health. Toluene residues are particularly concerning in medications taken by children or pregnant women.

Acetone: While generally less toxic than other solvents, acetone residues can cause respiratory irritation and nervous system effects, particularly in patients with existing respiratory or neurological conditions.

The Cumulative Solvent Problem

Patients taking multiple medications may be exposed to various solvent residues simultaneously, creating cumulative exposures that have never been studied for safety. Someone taking five different medications might consume residual amounts of methanol, benzene, toluene, and other industrial solvents daily, yet no regulatory agency evaluates the safety of these combined exposures.

The pharmaceutical industry argues that solvent residue levels are "negligible" and pose no health risks. However, these assessments typically consider individual solvents in isolation and don't account for cumulative exposure from multiple medications or increased vulnerability in sick patients whose bodies may be less able to eliminate toxic substances.

Cross-Contamination: When Medications Pollute Each Other

Modern pharmaceutical manufacturing often involves producing multiple different medications in the same facilities using shared equipment. This creates opportunities for cross-contamination where traces of one medication can end up in a completely different product, potentially exposing patients to unexpected drug interactions or allergic reactions.

Shared Equipment Contamination

Pharmaceutical companies often use the same mixing equipment, tableting machines, and packaging lines to produce different medications. Despite cleaning procedures between product runs, trace amounts of previous medications can remain on equipment and contaminate subsequent batches.

This cross-contamination can be particularly dangerous when potent medications like hormones, chemotherapy drugs, or psychiatric medications contaminate other products. Patients taking contaminated medications may experience unexpected side effects or drug interactions that healthcare providers struggle to explain.

Allergen Cross-Contamination

Cross-contamination becomes especially problematic when it involves common allergens. A medication that doesn't contain lactose as an ingredient might become contaminated with lactose residues from previous production runs of lactose-containing medications, triggering allergic reactions in lactose-intolerant patients.

Similarly, medications produced in facilities that also manufacture products containing peanuts, shellfish, or other common allergens may become cross-contaminated with trace amounts of these substances, potentially causing severe allergic reactions in sensitive patients.

API Cross-Contamination

Perhaps the most dangerous form of cross-contamination involves active pharmaceutical ingredients. When production equipment isn't adequately cleaned between different medications, patients may be exposed to trace amounts of drugs they're not supposed to be taking.

This type of contamination has led to cases where birth control pills were contaminated with blood pressure medications, causing dangerous drops in blood pressure in young women. Other incidents have involved contamination of children's medications with adult psychiatric drugs, causing serious adverse effects in pediatric patients.

The Valsartan Recall: Anatomy of a Contamination Crisis

The valsartan contamination crisis that began in 2018 provides a detailed case study of how pharmaceutical contamination develops, spreads, and ultimately affects millions of patients before being discovered and addressed. The crisis involved multiple types of contamination, numerous manufacturers, and regulatory failures that allowed dangerous medications to reach patients for years.

The Discovery

The valsartan crisis began when Novartis, the original developer of valsartan, was conducting routine testing and discovered NDMA contamination in generic versions of the medication produced by Zhejiang Huahai Pharmaceutical, a Chinese manufacturer that supplied valsartan to companies worldwide.

What made this discovery particularly alarming was the scale of contamination. The Chinese facility had been producing contaminated valsartan for years, supplying the contaminated ingredient to pharmaceutical companies around the world that used it in their own blood pressure medications. Millions of patients in dozens of countries had been consuming NDMA-contaminated blood pressure medications without knowing it.

The Manufacturing Process Problem

Investigation revealed that the NDMA contamination resulted from changes to the manufacturing process that Zhejiang Huahai had implemented to reduce costs and increase efficiency. The company had switched to a different solvent system and modified their chemical synthesis pathway without adequately testing for impurity formation.

The new manufacturing process created conditions that promoted NDMA formation as a byproduct of the chemical reactions used to produce valsartan. Instead of identifying and addressing this contamination, the company continued production and shipped contaminated products to customers worldwide.

Regulatory Failure

The valsartan crisis exposed serious gaps in regulatory oversight of pharmaceutical manufacturing. The Chinese facility producing the contaminated valsartan had been inspected by various regulatory agencies, including the FDA, but these inspections failed to identify the contamination problem.

The FDA's inspection reports from the facility showed that inspectors had identified various manufacturing deficiencies but had missed the fundamental process changes that were causing NDMA formation. This failure highlighted the inadequacy of current inspection procedures for detecting sophisticated contamination problems.

The Recall Cascade

Once NDMA contamination was discovered in valsartan, regulatory agencies around the world began testing other medications for similar contamination. This testing revealed widespread nitrosamine contamination affecting dozens of different medications from multiple manufacturers.

The recall process was chaotic and poorly coordinated, with different countries taking different approaches to managing contaminated medications. Some countries banned specific products immediately, while others allowed continued use while conducting "risk assessments" to determine whether the contamination posed significant health risks.

Patient Impact

The valsartan recalls affected millions of patients worldwide who had to switch to different blood pressure medications, often with different side effect profiles and effectiveness characteristics.

Many patients experienced blood pressure control problems during the transition period, and some suffered heart attacks or strokes that may have been related to inadequate blood pressure management during the medication switching process.

The psychological impact was equally significant, as patients lost confidence in the safety of their medications and began questioning whether other drugs they were taking might also be contaminated with cancer-causing chemicals.

The Cover-Up

Perhaps most disturbing were revelations that Zhejiang Huahai and other manufacturers had knowledge of contamination problems but failed to report them to regulators or customers. Internal company documents showed that the company had detected NDMA in their products but had conducted their own risk assessments concluding that the contamination levels were "acceptable."

This pattern of concealment was repeated at other facilities involved in nitrosamine contamination, suggesting that hiding contamination problems from regulators and customers is a widespread practice in the pharmaceutical industry.

The Ongoing Contamination Crisis

The valsartan recall was not an isolated incident but rather a window into systematic contamination problems that affect pharmaceutical manufacturing worldwide. Since 2018, contamination discoveries have continued at an alarming pace, affecting dozens of different medications and exposing millions of patients to preventable health risks.

Recent Contamination Events

The list of contaminated medications continues to grow, including:

Multiple blood pressure medications contaminated with various nitrosamines

Diabetes medications containing excessive NDMA levels

Heartburn medications contaminated with cancer-causing chemicals

Pain relievers containing heavy metal contamination

Antibiotics contaminated with industrial solvents

Generic drugs containing glass particles and metal fragments

Each contamination event follows a similar pattern: years of patient exposure before discovery, regulatory scrambling to assess risks and coordinate recalls, and pharmaceutical industry claims that the contamination poses minimal health risks.

The Testing Gap

One of the most troubling aspects of the ongoing contamination crisis is how many problems are discovered by accident rather than through systematic testing programs. Most contamination events are identified when manufacturers conduct voluntary testing or when academic researchers investigate specific compounds, not through routine regulatory oversight.

This reactive approach to contamination detection means that patients are essentially serving as unwitting test subjects for contaminated medications until problems become serious enough to trigger investigation and recall.

Protecting Yourself from Contamination

Given the current state of pharmaceutical contamination and regulatory oversight, patients who want to minimize their exposure to contaminated medications face significant challenges. However, there are steps you can take to reduce your risk:

Stay Informed About Recalls

The FDA maintains databases of drug recalls and safety alerts, but these resources require active monitoring by patients or healthcare providers. Subscribe to FDA safety alerts and regularly check recall databases, particularly for medications you take regularly.

Know Your Medication Sources

Ask pharmacists about the manufacturers of your medications and whether generic versions from specific companies have histories of contamination problems. Some manufacturers have better safety records than others, and this information can guide your medication choices.

Request Brand-Name Medications

While brand-name medications aren't immune to contamination, they typically have more stringent quality control systems and are less likely to be affected by the cost-cutting measures that often lead to contamination in generic manufacturing.

Monitor for Unusual Symptoms

Be alert to new or unusual symptoms that might be related to medication contamination rather than side effects of active ingredients. Unexplained health problems that develop after starting new medications or switching generic manufacturers may warrant investigation.

Advocate for Better Testing

Contact legislators and regulatory agencies to demand more systematic testing for contamination and stronger oversight of pharmaceutical manufacturing, particularly for facilities in countries with less stringent environmental and safety regulations.

The Cover-Up Culture

Perhaps the most disturbing aspect of pharmaceutical contamination isn't the contamination itself—it's the systematic culture of concealment that allows dangerous products to reach patients while companies conduct internal risk assessments to determine whether fixing the problems is commercially viable.

Internal Risk-Benefit Analysis

Documents obtained through litigation have revealed that pharmaceutical companies routinely conduct cost-benefit analyses when contamination is discovered. These internal assessments weigh the cost of fixing contamination problems against the potential financial liability from lawsuits and regulatory action.

In many cases, companies conclude that it's more profitable to continue selling contaminated products while monitoring for regulatory action than to halt production and fix manufacturing problems. These calculations treat patient health as just another cost factor in business decisions, with human lives reduced to statistical probabilities and financial projections.

The Regulatory Notification Gap

Even when companies discover contamination, they often delay reporting to regulatory agencies while conducting their own investigations. This delay can last months or years, during which time contaminated products continue reaching patients.

The pharmaceutical industry argues that immediate reporting of every potential contamination would create unnecessary alarm and disrupt medication supply chains. Critics point out that this approach prioritizes industry convenience over patient safety, allowing companies to determine privately whether contamination poses "significant" risks before involving regulators.

Legal Strategy Considerations

Internal company documents show that legal departments play major roles in contamination response decisions. Companies often prioritize minimizing legal liability over maximizing patient safety, consulting with attorneys before taking any action that might be interpreted as admission of fault.

This legal-first approach to contamination can delay remediation efforts and limit the scope of recalls to minimize financial exposure. Companies may recall only specific batches known to be contaminated rather than all potentially affected products, leaving patients uncertain about whether their medications are safe.

The International Manufacturing Shell Game

The globalization of pharmaceutical manufacturing has created a complex web of subsidiaries, contractors, and distributors that makes it nearly impossible to trace contamination back to its source or hold responsible parties accountable for patient harm.

Contract Manufacturing Complexity

Many pharmaceutical companies no longer manufacture their own products, instead contracting with specialized manufacturing facilities around the world. These contract manufacturers often produce medications for multiple companies simultaneously, creating opportunities for contamination to affect numerous different branded products.

When contamination occurs in contract manufacturing facilities, responsibility becomes diffused among multiple parties—the contract manufacturer, the pharmaceutical company that owns the product, and various intermediary distributors and suppliers. This complexity makes it difficult for patients to determine who's responsible for their contaminated medications and how to seek compensation for health damages.

Subsidiary Shield Strategies

Pharmaceutical companies often structure their overseas manufacturing operations through complex networks of subsidiaries and joint ventures that provide legal protection when contamination problems arise. These corporate structures can shield parent companies from liability while making it difficult for patients and regulators to identify responsible parties.

When contamination scandals emerge, companies often blame foreign subsidiaries or suppliers, claiming limited oversight and control over manufacturing processes they actually direct and profit from. This corporate shell game allows companies to benefit from cheap overseas manufacturing while avoiding responsibility for the safety problems that result.

Supply Chain Opacity

The complexity of modern pharmaceutical supply chains means that companies can credibly claim ignorance about contamination sources while continuing to profit from potentially dangerous products. Raw materials may pass through multiple intermediaries before reaching final manufacturers, creating opportunities for contamination introduction at numerous points in the supply chain.

This opacity serves pharmaceutical companies' interests by providing plausible deniability when contamination occurs, but it leaves patients and regulators unable to assess risks or implement effective oversight of manufacturing processes.

The Regulatory Whack-a-Mole Problem

Current approaches to pharmaceutical contamination treat each incident as an isolated problem to be fixed rather than recognizing the systematic issues that make contamination inevitable under current manufacturing and oversight practices.

Reactive Rather Than Preventive

Regulatory agencies typically respond to contamination by issuing recalls and conducting investigations, but they rarely implement systematic changes that would prevent similar problems from occurring in other facilities or with various products.

This reactive approach means that each contamination incident represents a failure of the regulatory system rather than evidence that the system is working to protect patients. By the time contamination is discovered and addressed, patients have already been exposed to potentially harmful substances for months or years.

The Inspection Theater

FDA inspections of pharmaceutical facilities often follow predictable schedules and focus on documentation review rather than actual testing for contamination. Facilities receive advance notice of inspections, allowing them to temporarily modify practices or hide evidence of contamination problems.

Even when inspections identify manufacturing deficiencies, the follow-up process is often slow and bureaucratic, allowing facilities to continue operating while appeals and corrective action plans wind through regulatory channels. This system prioritizes maintaining medication supply chains over ensuring medication safety.

Jurisdictional Limitations

The global nature of pharmaceutical manufacturing creates jurisdictional problems that limit regulatory effectiveness. FDA authority over foreign facilities is limited by international law and diplomatic considerations, making it difficult to implement meaningful oversight of overseas manufacturing operations.

When contamination occurs in foreign facilities, regulatory responses often depend on cooperation from foreign governments and manufacturers rather than direct enforcement authority. This dependency relationship gives foreign manufacturers significant leverage to resist regulatory demands and delay remediation efforts.

The Patient Information Blackout

One of the most troubling aspects of pharmaceutical contamination is how little information patients receive about the risks they face and the contamination events that affect their medications.

Recall Communication Failures

When contaminated medications are recalled, patient notification is often inadequate and confusing. Recalls may be announced through obscure regulatory websites and technical publications that patients never see, leaving them unaware that their medications have been deemed unsafe.

Even when patients learn about recalls affecting their medications, the information provided is often technical and difficult to understand. Patients may not know whether specific lot numbers or dates affect their medications, or what actions they should take to protect their health.

Healthcare Provider Information Gaps

Healthcare providers often know little more than patients about contamination events affecting medications they prescribe. Pharmaceutical companies typically provide minimal information to healthcare providers about contamination incidents, focusing on technical details rather than practical guidance for patient care.

This information gap means that healthcare providers can't adequately counsel patients about contamination risks or help them make informed decisions about medication alternatives when contamination occurs.

Long-Term Health Monitoring Absence

Perhaps most troubling is the complete absence of systematic monitoring for health effects in patients who have been exposed to contaminated medications. When contamination is discovered, regulatory agencies and pharmaceutical companies typically conduct theoretical risk assessments rather than actual health monitoring of affected patients.

This approach means that the real health consequences of pharmaceutical contamination remain largely unknown, allowing companies and regulators to claim that contamination poses minimal risks without any empirical evidence to support these claims.

The contamination crisis in pharmaceutical manufacturing represents one of the most serious threats to medication safety in modern history. Millions of patients have been exposed to cancer-causing chemicals, toxic metals, and industrial solvents through medications they trusted to improve their health. Until we demand fundamental reforms in manufacturing oversight and quality control, patients will continue to serve as unwitting test subjects for contaminated medications that prioritize cost reduction over safety.

The next time you take a prescription medication, remember that it may contain not just the active ingredient you need, but also cancer-causing chemicals, toxic metals, and industrial solvents that have no business being in medicines. The pharmaceutical industry's approach to contamination treats patient safety as a cost to be minimized rather than a priority to be protected and only sustained public pressure will force the changes necessary to ensure that medications heal rather than harm.

Chapter 7: Generic vs. Brand Name Reality

The first time I experienced the difference between brand-name and generic medications wasn't through any scientific study or medical journal—it was through my own body's violent reaction to what was supposed to be an identical medication. After years of successfully taking a brand-name pain medication following one of my surgeries, my insurance company mandated that I switch to the generic version to save costs. "It's exactly the same," the pharmacist assured me. "Just a different manufacturer."

Within three days of making the switch, I was experiencing severe digestive problems, headaches, and symptoms I'd never had with the brand-name version. When I called my doctor, he initially dismissed my concerns, suggesting it was psychological or coincidental. It took several weeks of advocacy and documentation before he agreed to prescribe the brand-name version again, during which time my symptoms disappeared completely.

This experience taught me that the pharmaceutical industry's claim that generic medications are "identical" to brand-name drugs is one of the most dangerous myths in modern medicine. While generics may contain the same active ingredient, they can differ dramatically in their inactive ingredients, manufacturing processes, quality control standards, and ultimately, their effects on patients' bodies.

The generic drug system in America is built on a regulatory fiction—the idea that medications with the same active ingredient will have identical effects in patients, regardless of how they're manufactured or what other chemicals they contain. This fiction serves the monetary interests of insurance companies and generic manufacturers while exposing patients to unnecessary risks and unpredictable medication effects.

The Bioequivalence Deception

The foundation of generic drug approval in the United States rests on the concept of "bioequivalence"—the idea that generic medications deliver the same amount of active ingredient to patients' bloodstreams as brand-name drugs. What most patients and even many healthcare providers don't understand is that this bioequivalence standard allows for significant variations in how medications behave in the body.

The 80-125% Rule

The FDA's bioequivalence standard allows generic medications to deliver anywhere from 80% to 125% of the active ingredient compared to the brand-name version. This means that switching from a brand-name drug to a generic could result in receiving 20% less active ingredient, or switching between different generic manufacturers could create a 45% difference in drug exposure (from 80% to 125%).

To put this in perspective, imagine if your morning coffee could legally contain anywhere from 80% to 125% of the caffeine listed on the label. Some days you'd feel under-caffeinated, other days you'd be jittery and overstimulated, yet the manufacturer could claim all variations were "equivalent" to regular coffee.

For medications with narrow therapeutic windows—where slight changes in dose can mean the difference between therapeutic effect and toxicity—this 45% variation range can be the difference between effective treatment and dangerous side effects or treatment failure.

The Statistical Shell Game

The bioequivalence testing process itself masks significant variations in individual patient responses. The FDA requires generic manufacturers to demonstrate that the average bioequivalence of their product falls within the 80-125% range when tested in healthy volunteers, typically young adults without the medical conditions the medications are designed to treat.

This average-based approach can hide substantial individual variations. A generic medication might pass bioequivalence testing even if 20% of test subjects experienced bioequivalence outside the acceptable range, as long as the overall average falls within FDA limits. Individual patients who respond differently to generic formulations are essentially statistical outliers whose experiences are dismissed as irrelevant to regulatory approval.

The Healthy Volunteer Problem

Perhaps more problematic is that bioequivalence testing is conducted in healthy volunteers rather than patients with the conditions the medications are designed to treat. A generic heart medication might show acceptable bioequivalence in healthy 25-year-olds but behave very differently in 70-year-olds with heart disease, kidney problems, and compromised circulation.

This testing approach ignores the reality that sick patients often process medications differently than healthy individuals. Changes in stomach acidity, digestive function, kidney clearance, and liver metabolism that accompany illness can all affect how medications are absorbed and metabolized, potentially making bioequivalence data from healthy volunteers irrelevant to actual patient populations.

The Inactive Ingredient Wild Card

While generic medications must contain the same active ingredient as brand-name drugs, they can use completely different inactive ingredients, creating medications that may behave very differently in patients' bodies despite containing identical active compounds.

Formulation Freedom

Generic manufacturers have complete freedom to choose their own excipients, fillers, binders, coatings, and other inactive ingredients, as long as these substances are on the FDA's list of approved pharmaceutical ingredients. This means that a generic medication might contain entirely different allergens, preservatives, and chemical additives than the brand-name version.

For patients with food allergies, chemical sensitivities, or dietary restrictions, switching to a generic medication can be like playing Russian roulette with their health. A patient who has successfully taken a lactose-free brand-name medication for years might suddenly experience severe digestive problems when switched to a generic version that uses lactose as a primary filler.

Dissolution and Absorption Differences

The inactive ingredients in medications don't just serve as inert packaging—they actively control how quickly medications dissolve, how completely they're absorbed, and how consistently they deliver active ingredients to the bloodstream. Different excipient systems can create dramatically different absorption patterns even when the same amount of active ingredient is present.

A generic medication might dissolve much faster than the brand-name version, creating higher peak blood levels that cause side effects, or it might dissolve more slowly, resulting in inadequate therapeutic levels. These differences can occur even when the generic version passes bioequivalence testing, because bioequivalence is measured as total drug exposure over 24 hours rather than the pattern of drug delivery throughout that period.

The Coating Controversy

Many modern medications use sophisticated coating systems to control drug release, protect active ingredients from stomach acid, or mask unpleasant tastes. Generic manufacturers often use different coating materials and techniques, potentially creating medications that behave very differently despite containing identical active ingredients.

Enteric-coated medications designed to bypass the stomach and dissolve in the intestines are particularly problematic. Different coating materials may dissolve at different pH levels or respond differently to digestive conditions, potentially causing medications to release their contents in the wrong part of the digestive system.

Quality Control: The Manufacturing Divide

The quality control standards and manufacturing practices used by generic drug manufacturers often differ significantly from those employed by brand-name pharmaceutical companies, creating opportunities for batch-to-batch variation and quality problems that can affect patient safety and medication effectiveness.

Manufacturing Scale and Sophistication

Brand-name pharmaceutical companies typically invest heavily in state-of-the-art manufacturing facilities with sophisticated quality control systems, automated production lines, and extensive testing protocols. These companies have strong financial incentives to maintain consistent quality because their brand reputation depends on product reliability.

Generic manufacturers, competing primarily on price, often operate with much smaller profit margins that limit their ability to invest in advanced manufacturing systems. Many generic manufacturing facilities, particularly those in developing countries, use older equipment and less sophisticated quality control procedures than their brand-name counterparts.

Batch-to-Batch Variation

Generic medications often show much greater batch-to-batch variation than brand-name drugs, meaning that the medication you receive this month might be noticeably different from the same medication you received last month, even from the same manufacturer.

This variation can occur in active ingredient potency, dissolution rates, physical characteristics, and inactive ingredient composition. Patients taking generic medications may experience fluctuating effectiveness or side effects that correspond to different manufacturing batches, creating an unpredictable treatment experience.

Supply Chain Complexity

Generic manufacturers often source their raw materials and active ingredients from multiple suppliers, switching between sources based on price and availability. This supply chain complexity can introduce variation in medication quality that doesn't exist with brand-name drugs, which typically maintain more stable supplier relationships.

Changes in raw material suppliers can affect everything from active ingredient purity to inactive ingredient composition, potentially creating medications that differ significantly from previous batches even when manufactured by the same company using the same formulation.

The Pharmacy Switching Problem

Perhaps the most problematic aspect of generic medication use is the customary practice of pharmacies switching between different generic manufacturers based on their wholesale purchasing agreements, often without informing patients or healthcare providers about these changes.

The Monthly Manufacturer Roulette

Most pharmacies purchase generic medications from whichever manufacturer offers the lowest price during their purchasing cycle, which may change monthly or quarterly. This means that patients taking generic medications may unknowingly switch between different manufacturers multiple times per year, each time receiving medications with different inactive ingredients, manufacturing processes, and quality control standards.

For patients with chronic conditions requiring stable medication levels, this constant switching can create a therapeutic roller coaster of varying effectiveness and side effects. A patient might achieve good symptom control with one manufacturer's generic, only to experience breakthrough symptoms or new side effects when their pharmacy switches to a different manufacturer.

The Information Gap

Most patients are never informed when their pharmacy switches generic manufacturers, and many pharmacies don't maintain records that would allow them to identify which manufacturer supplied specific prescriptions. This makes it nearly impossible for patients and healthcare providers to identify patterns connecting symptoms with specific generic formulations.

When patients experience problems with generic medications, healthcare providers often attribute these issues to disease progression, drug tolerance, or other factors rather than recognizing that the patient may be responding to a different formulation of the same medication.

Insurance Formulary Restrictions

Insurance companies often mandate specific generic manufacturers to maximize their cost savings, preventing patients from requesting alternative generic formulations even when they experience problems with particular manufacturers. This system prioritizes insurance company profits over patient health outcomes.

Patients who experience problems with mandated generic formulations may be forced to pay out-of-pocket for brand-name medications or alternative generic manufacturers, creating a two-tiered system where medication quality depends on financial resources rather than medical necessity.

When Switching Becomes Dangerous

For certain types of medications and patient populations, switching between brand-name and generic formulations or between different generic manufacturers can create serious health risks that may not become apparent until significant harm has occurred.

Narrow Therapeutic Index Medications

Medications with narrow therapeutic indexes—where minor changes in blood levels can mean the difference between therapeutic effect and dangerous toxicity—are particularly problematic for generic substitution. These medications include blood thinners, anti-seizure drugs, heart rhythm medications, and thyroid hormones.

For patients taking warfarin, a blood-thinning medication, even small variations in bioequivalence can result in dangerous blood clotting or life-threatening bleeding. Switching between different generic warfarin manufacturers has been associated with emergency hospital admissions for bleeding complications and stroke.

Anti-seizure medications present similar risks, as variations in bioequivalence can trigger breakthrough seizures in patients whose epilepsy was previously well-controlled. The consequences of seizure breakthrough can include serious injuries, loss of driving privileges, and psychological trauma that affects patients' quality of life for months or years.

Cardiovascular Medication Risks

Heart rhythm medications and blood pressure drugs are particularly sensitive to formulation differences because cardiovascular patients often have compromised circulation and altered drug metabolism that can amplify the effects of bioequivalence variations.

Patients taking medication for irregular heart rhythms may experience dangerous arrhythmias when switched to generic formulations with different dissolution or absorption characteristics. Blood pressure patients may experience dangerous spikes or drops in blood pressure that increase their risk of heart attack, stroke, or kidney damage.

Psychiatric Medication Stability

Psychiatric medications often require months of careful dose adjustment to achieve stable symptom control, making patients particularly vulnerable to the effects of switching between different formulations. Minor changes in bioequivalence can destabilize patients' mental health, potentially triggering relapses of depression, anxiety, or other psychiatric conditions.

The consequences of psychiatric medication instability extend beyond the patients themselves, affecting their families, employers, and communities. A patient whose depression is destabilized by a generic medication switch might lose their job, damage relationships, or experience suicidal thoughts that require emergency intervention.

Pediatric and Elderly Vulnerability

Children and elderly patients are particularly vulnerable to the effects of medication switching because their bodies process drugs differently than healthy adults. Children's developing metabolic systems and elderly patients' declining organ function can amplify the effects of bioequivalence variations.

Elderly patients taking multiple medications face compound risks when several generic medications are switched simultaneously, potentially creating dangerous drug interactions or cumulative effects that wouldn't occur with stable brand-name formulations.

The Economic Pressure Cooker

The financial pressures driving generic medication use create systematic biases that prioritize cost savings over patient safety, often trapping patients in systems that expose them to unnecessary health risks.

Insurance Company Mandates

Health insurance companies routinely mandate generic substitution to reduce their medication costs, often implementing policies that make it difficult or impossible for patients to access brand-name medications even when medical necessity is documented.

These mandates are typically implemented by insurance company administrators and pharmacists rather than physicians who understand the medical complexities of medication switching. The result is a system where financial considerations override medical judgment in medication selection.

Pharmacy Benefit Manager Conflicts

Pharmacy Benefit Managers (PBMs) that negotiate drug prices for insurance companies often have financial relationships with generic manufacturers that create conflicts of interest in formulary decisions. These companies may promote specific generic manufacturers based on financial kickbacks rather than quality or patient outcomes.

The complexity of PBM relationships with pharmaceutical manufacturers makes it nearly impossible for patients and healthcare providers to understand the financial incentives driving medication selection decisions.

Healthcare Provider Pressures

Healthcare providers face increasing pressure from insurance companies, hospitals, and practice administrators to prescribe generic medications regardless of medical considerations. Physicians who frequently prescribe brand-name medications may face scrutiny or financial penalties that discourage them from prioritizing patient safety over cost considerations.

This pressure can compromise the physician-patient relationship and interfere with medical decision-making, creating situations where healthcare providers feel compelled to recommend medications based on administrative convenience rather than optimal patient care.

The Quality Assurance Illusion

The regulatory systems designed to ensure generic medication quality often create an illusion of oversight while failing to detect problems that affect real-world patient outcomes.

Inspection Frequency Gaps

Generic manufacturing facilities are inspected much less frequently than brand-name facilities, often going years between FDA inspections. Many overseas generic manufacturers have never been inspected by American regulators, despite supplying medications to millions of American patients.

When inspections do occur, they typically focus on documentation and procedures rather than actual product testing, meaning that quality problems affecting finished medications may not be detected even during supposedly thorough regulatory reviews.

Testing Protocol Limitations

The testing protocols used to verify generic medication quality focus primarily on active ingredient content and basic dissolution testing, often missing problems with inactive ingredients, contamination, or manufacturing defects that can significantly affect patient outcomes.

These limited testing protocols create opportunities for quality problems to reach patients while still meeting regulatory requirements, undermining confidence in the generic approval and monitoring systems.

Post-Market Surveillance Deficiencies

Unlike brand-name medications, which are closely monitored by their manufacturers for adverse events and quality problems, generic medications often have minimal post-market surveillance systems. When patients experience problems with generic medications, these issues may not be systematically collected or analyzed to identify patterns indicating quality problems.

This surveillance gap means that quality problems with generic medications may affect thousands of patients before being identified and addressed if they're ever identified at all.

Protecting Yourself in the Generic Maze

Given the current realities of generic medication quality and regulation, patients who want to minimize their risks while still accessing affordable medications need strategies for navigating the complex generic medication landscape.

Document Your Medication Sources

Keep detailed records of which manufacturers produce your generic medications and track any changes in symptoms or side effects that correspond to manufacturer switches. This information can help you and your healthcare provider identify problematic formulations and request alternatives.

Many pharmacies don't maintain records of which manufacturers supplied specific prescriptions, so patient documentation may be the only way to identify connections between symptoms and specific generic formulations.

Request Manufacturer Consistency

Ask your pharmacy to maintain consistency with generic manufacturers whenever possible, even if it means paying slightly higher costs for specific formulations. Many pharmacies can order medications from specific manufacturers if patients request this service.

For critical medications like blood thinners, anti-seizure drugs, or heart medications, manufacturer consistency may be essential for maintaining stable therapeutic effects and avoiding dangerous complications.

Know Your Insurance Options

Understand your insurance company's procedures for requesting brand-name medications when medical necessity can be documented. Many insurance plans have appeal processes that allow coverage of brand-name medications when patients experience problems with generic alternatives.

Work with your healthcare provider to document any adverse effects or therapeutic failures associated with generic medications, as this documentation may be required for insurance appeals.

Advocate for Better Regulation

Support legislative and regulatory efforts to improve generic medication quality standards, increase inspection frequency for generic manufacturers, and require better disclosure of formulation differences between generic and brand-name medications.

Contact representatives to demand stronger oversight of generic medication quality and better protection for patients who experience problems with generic formulations.

The generic medication system in America represents a massive uncontrolled experiment in pharmaceutical cost-cutting that treats patients as interchangeable test subjects rather than individuals with unique medical needs and sensitivities. While generic medications can provide important cost savings and access benefits, the current system's emphasis on price over quality creates unnecessary risks that affect millions of patients daily.

Until we acknowledge that identical active ingredients don't guarantee identical patient outcomes, and until we implement quality standards that prioritize patient safety over cost savings, patients will continue to serve as unwitting participants in a pharmaceutical lottery where medication effectiveness and safety depend more on manufacturing economics than medical science.

The next time your pharmacy tells you that a generic medication is "exactly the same" as the brand-name version, remember that this claim ignores everything we know about how inactive ingredients, manufacturing processes, and quality control standards affect medication performance in real patients. In a rational healthcare system, medication substitution decisions would be based on documented therapeutic equivalence rather than chemical similarity, but we don't live in that system yet.

Chapter 8: The Inspection Game

When I first learned about the global pharmaceutical manufacturing crisis, my immediate assumption was that the FDA must be conducting rigorous, surprise inspections to catch contamination and quality problems before they reach patients. I imagined teams of eagle-eyed investigators swooping into facilities unannounced, armed with sophisticated testing equipment and the authority to shut down operations immediately if they found safety violations.

The reality couldn't be more different.

What I discovered through months of research into FDA inspection practices is a system so compromised by advance notice, diplomatic constraints, and bureaucratic limitations that it functions more like theater than actual oversight. Pharmaceutical manufacturers receive advance warning of most inspections, allowing them to temporarily clean up operations, hide evidence of problems, and present sanitized versions of their manufacturing processes to regulators.

Even when inspectors do identify serious safety violations, the enforcement mechanisms available to them are so slow and cumbersome that contaminated or dangerous medications can continue reaching patients for months or years while appeals and corrective action plans wind through bureaucratic channels. The inspection system gives both regulators and the public a false sense of security while failing to protect patients from the very problems it's supposed to prevent.

The Advance Notice Problem

Perhaps the most fundamental flaw in pharmaceutical inspection practices is the routine provision of advance notice to facilities being inspected. Unlike restaurant health inspections or workplace safety visits, which are typically conducted without warning to observe actual operating conditions, pharmaceutical facility inspections are usually scheduled weeks or months in advance.

The Diplomatic Dance

For overseas facilities, inspection scheduling becomes a complex diplomatic process involving multiple governments, regulatory agencies, and corporate entities. The FDA must formally request permission from foreign governments to conduct inspections, provide detailed information about the scope and timing of their visits, and coordinate with local regulatory authorities who may have their own relationships with the facilities being inspected.

This diplomatic process can take months, during which facility managers have ample time to prepare for inspection visits. Documents can be organized, problematic employees can be reassigned or trained, temporary quality control measures can be implemented, and physical evidence of problems can be removed or concealed.

The Preparation Advantage

Pharmaceutical companies have turned advance notice into a competitive advantage, developing sophisticated "inspection readiness" programs that allow them to quickly transform their operations when regulatory visits are scheduled. These programs often include:

Temporary hiring of additional quality control staff to improve inspection metrics

Implementation of enhanced cleaning and maintenance procedures that aren't maintained year-round

Preparation of carefully curated document sets that highlight positive aspects while concealing problems

Training programs that teach employees how to respond to inspector questions in ways that minimize regulatory concerns

Temporary suspension of problematic manufacturing processes or product lines during inspection periods

The result is that inspectors often see idealized versions of manufacturing operations rather than the day-to-day reality of how medications are actually produced.

The Clean-Up Window

The advance notice system creates a "clean-up window" that allows facilities to address obvious problems before inspectors arrive while leaving systemic issues unchanged. A facility might temporarily upgrade its water purification systems, implement additional testing protocols, or address documentation deficiencies without making fundamental changes to manufacturing processes that create ongoing quality risks.

This superficial remediation gives inspectors a false impression of facility capabilities while ensuring that problems will resurface once the inspection is complete and normal operations resume.

The Access Limitations

Even when FDA inspectors arrive at pharmaceutical facilities, their access is often limited by corporate policies, security restrictions, and legal constraints that prevent them from observing actual manufacturing operations or accessing complete information about production processes.

The Guided Tour Approach

Most pharmaceutical facility inspections follow a carefully orchestrated tour format where company representatives' control which areas inspectors can visit, which employees they can interview, and which documents they can review. This guided tour approach ensures that inspectors see only what companies want them to see.

Inspectors may be shown state-of-the-art quality control laboratories while being denied access to actual production areas where contamination or quality problems are occurring. They might be permitted to review selected batch records while being told that other records are unavailable due to proprietary concerns or legal restrictions.

Trade Secret Barriers

Pharmaceutical companies routinely invoke trade secret protections to limit inspector access to manufacturing processes, formulations, and quality control data. While some information legitimately deserves protection from competitors, the trade secret shield is often used to hide problems rather than protect intellectual property.

Inspectors may be told that specific manufacturing processes can't be observed because they involve proprietary techniques, or that certain quality control data can't be shared because it contains competitive information. These restrictions make it impossible for inspectors to fully evaluate facility operations or identify potential safety problems.

Time and Resource Constraints

FDA inspections are typically scheduled for just a few days, which is insufficient time to thoroughly evaluate complex pharmaceutical manufacturing operations. Inspectors must attempt to assess months or years of manufacturing activity through document review and brief facility tours, making it easy for companies to conceal ongoing problems.

The limited inspection timeline also creates opportunities for facilities to temporarily modify their operations during inspection periods. Problematic manufacturing processes can be suspended, problem employees can be reassigned, and enhanced quality control measures can be implemented just long enough to satisfy inspector requirements.

The Documentation Deception

Modern pharmaceutical facility inspections rely heavily on document review rather than direct observation of manufacturing processes, creating opportunities for companies to present misleading information while concealing actual operational problems.

The Paper Trail Illusion

Pharmaceutical companies maintain extensive documentation systems that create an illusion of rigorous quality control while potentially masking significant operational problems. These documentation systems often include:

Batch production records that may be selectively edited or retroactively modified

Quality control testing data that may exclude failed tests or anomalous results

Standard operating procedures that describe idealized processes rather than actual practices

Training records that document required training completion without verifying actual competency

Corrective action reports that may minimize problems or claim resolution without implementing effective changes

Inspectors reviewing these documents may develop confidence in facility operations based on paperwork that doesn't reflect manufacturing reality.

The Selective Disclosure Problem

Companies have significant discretion in determining which documents to present to inspectors and how to organize information to minimize regulatory concerns. Problematic test results might be buried in voluminous data sets, equipment maintenance problems might be categorized as "routine" rather than safety-related, and customer complaints might be dismissed as user error rather than product defects.

This selective disclosure allows companies to technically comply with inspection requirements while ensuring that inspectors don't develop a complete picture of facility operations or safety problems.

The Retroactive Revision Strategy

Some facilities engage in retroactive revision of documentation when they learn that inspections are scheduled. Batch records might be "corrected" to eliminate evidence of deviations from standard procedures, quality control data might be re-analyzed using different criteria to improve results, and employee training records might be updated to demonstrate compliance with current requirements.

These retroactive revisions can make it appear that facilities have been operating in compliance with regulations when they've actually been experiencing ongoing quality problems.

The Enforcement Theater

Even when FDA inspectors identify serious safety violations during facility inspections, the enforcement mechanisms available to address these problems are so slow and bureaucratic that they often fail to protect patients from ongoing risks.

The Warning Letter Ritual

The FDA's primary enforcement tool for addressing inspection violations is the warning letter—a formal notification that describes problems identified during inspections and requests corrective action from facilities. These letters are supposed to initiate an escalating enforcement process that can ultimately lead to facility shutdowns and criminal prosecution.

In practice, warning letters have become a bureaucratic ritual that allows both companies and regulators to claim they're addressing safety problems without implementing meaningful changes. Companies typically respond to warning letters with detailed "corrective action plans" that promise to fix identified problems, often without actually changing the practices that caused the violations.

The Appeal and Delay Strategy

Pharmaceutical companies have developed sophisticated strategies for appealing inspection findings and delaying enforcement actions while continuing to operate facilities with known safety problems. These strategies often include:

Challenging inspector findings through formal appeal processes that can take months or years to resolve

Implementing superficial corrective actions that address inspection observations without fixing underlying problems

Hiring former FDA officials as consultants to help navigate regulatory challenges and minimize enforcement risks

Threatening to cease production of critical medications if enforcement actions proceed, creating pressure on regulators to accept minimal compliance measures

The Regulatory Capture Problem

The pharmaceutical industry's influence over FDA inspection and enforcement practices extends beyond formal lobbying to include the "revolving door" between regulatory agencies and industry employers. Many FDA officials responsible for inspection oversight later take high-paying jobs with pharmaceutical companies, creating conflicts of interest that may influence their regulatory decisions.

This revolving door relationship means that FDA officials may be reluctant to pursue aggressive enforcement actions against companies that might later become their employers. The result is a regulatory culture that tends to give pharmaceutical companies the benefit of the doubt and accept minimal compliance measures rather than demanding fundamental operational changes.

The International Inspection Crisis

The globalization of pharmaceutical manufacturing has created inspection challenges that the FDA is fundamentally unprepared to address, leaving millions of patients dependent on medications produced in facilities that receive minimal or no regulatory oversight.

The Scale Problem

The FDA's Office of Global Policy and Strategy employs approximately 200 investigators responsible for inspecting over 3,000 foreign pharmaceutical facilities across dozens of countries. This means that the average foreign facility manufacturing medications for American patients can expect an FDA inspection perhaps once every 15 years, if at all.

Many facilities that supply critical medications to American patients have never been inspected by FDA investigators, despite operating for years or decades. The scale mismatch between regulatory resources and oversight responsibilities makes meaningful inspection coverage impossible under current staffing levels.

The Diplomatic Constraints

FDA authority over foreign pharmaceutical facilities is severely limited by international law and diplomatic considerations. The agency cannot conduct surprise inspections of foreign facilities, cannot compel cooperation from foreign companies, and cannot directly enforce American safety standards in other countries.

When foreign facilities refuse to cooperate with inspection requests or deny FDA investigators access to manufacturing areas, the agency's primary recourse is to ban imports from those facilities. However, import bans can create medication shortages that affect patient care, creating pressure on regulators to accept minimal compliance rather than protect patient safety.

The Cultural and Language Barriers

FDA inspectors conducting overseas inspections often face significant cultural and language barriers that limit their ability to effectively evaluate facility operations. These barriers include:

Language differences that make it difficult to communicate with facility employees or understand documentation

Cultural practices that may emphasize saving face or avoiding conflict rather than honest disclosure of problems

Different regulatory traditions that may not emphasize the same safety priorities as American standards

Local government relationships that may influence facility cooperation with American investigators

These barriers create opportunities for facilities to conceal problems from American inspectors while technically complying with inspection requirements.

The Technology Inspection Gap

Modern pharmaceutical manufacturing increasingly relies on sophisticated technology and automation systems that FDA inspectors often lack the expertise to evaluate, creating blind spots in inspection coverage that can miss critical safety problems.

The Expertise Mismatch

FDA inspectors are typically trained in traditional pharmaceutical manufacturing techniques and may lack the specialized knowledge needed to evaluate modern automated production systems, computerized quality control processes, or advanced analytical testing equipment.

This expertise gap means that inspectors may be unable to identify problems with computer-controlled manufacturing processes, may not understand how to evaluate the integrity of electronic data systems, or may miss safety issues related to software malfunctions or programming errors.

The Data Integrity Problem

Modern pharmaceutical manufacturing generates enormous amounts of electronic data that can be easily manipulated, deleted, or selectively presented to inspectors. Companies may present favorable data subsets while concealing problematic results, or they may use sophisticated data management systems to hide evidence of quality control failures.

FDA inspectors often lack the forensic data analysis skills needed to detect data manipulation or to identify patterns that might indicate systematic quality problems. This limitation allows companies to present misleading information while technically complying with inspection requirements.

The Automation Oversight Challenge

Automated pharmaceutical manufacturing systems can operate with minimal human oversight, potentially allowing quality problems to persist for extended periods without detection. These systems may produce thousands of medication doses with identical defects before problems are identified and corrected.

FDA inspectors evaluating automated systems may see only summary reports of system performance rather than detailed logs that would reveal intermittent problems or systematic errors. This limited visibility makes it difficult to assess the actual quality and safety of medications produced by automated systems.

The Inspection Frequency Illusion

Public confidence in pharmaceutical safety often rests on the assumption that manufacturing facilities are regularly inspected and closely monitored by regulatory authorities. The reality is that most facilities receive inspections so infrequently that they provide little meaningful oversight of ongoing operations.

The Domestic Inspection Schedule

Even domestic pharmaceutical facilities are inspected relatively infrequently, with the FDA targeting inspections every two to three years for most facilities. This inspection frequency means that facilities can operate with significant quality problems for years between regulatory visits.

The scheduled nature of most domestic inspections also allows facilities to prepare extensively for inspector visits, implementing temporary improvements that may not reflect normal operating conditions.

The Risk-Based Inspection Myth

The FDA claims to use "risk-based" inspection scheduling that prioritizes facilities with higher safety risks or histories of compliance problems. However, the agency's risk assessment processes often rely on information provided by the facilities themselves, creating opportunities for companies to minimize their apparent risk profiles.

Facilities with serious quality problems may avoid frequent inspection by maintaining good documentation systems, responding promptly to regulatory communications, and avoiding obvious compliance violations that would trigger increased oversight.

The Post-Inspection Follow-Up Gap

One of the most significant weaknesses in the inspection system is the limited follow-up conducted after inspections identify problems. Facilities that receive warning letters or other enforcement actions may not be re-inspected for years, allowing them to revert to problematic practices once regulatory attention has moved elsewhere.

This follow-up gap means that corrective actions implemented in response to inspection findings may be temporary measures designed to satisfy regulators rather than permanent improvements to manufacturing operations.

The Whistleblower Suppression System

Perhaps most troubling is the pharmaceutical industry's systematic suppression of employee whistleblowers who might expose safety problems to regulatory authorities or the public.

The Non-Disclosure Web

Pharmaceutical companies routinely require employees to sign extensive non-disclosure agreements that limit their ability to report safety concerns to external authorities. These agreements often include severe financial penalties for employees who violate confidentiality requirements, creating powerful disincentives for reporting quality problems.

Employees who discover contamination, quality control failures, or other safety problems may be legally prevented from reporting these issues to the FDA, state health agencies, or patient advocacy groups.

The Retaliation Reality

Employees who do report safety concerns often face retaliation from their employers, including termination, demotion, transfer to undesirable positions, or blacklisting within the pharmaceutical industry. These retaliation practices effectively silence potential whistleblowers and prevent safety information from reaching regulatory authorities.

The pharmaceutical industry's tight-knit nature means that employees who gain reputations as whistleblowers may find it difficult to obtain employment elsewhere in the industry, creating long-term career consequences for those who prioritize patient safety over corporate loyalty.

The Legal Protection Gaps

While federal and state laws theoretically protect pharmaceutical industry whistleblowers, these protections are often inadequate in practice. Employees may face years of legal battles to prove retaliation, during which time they may be unemployed and facing financial hardship.

The complexity and cost of pursuing whistleblower protection claims often deter employees from reporting safety concerns, allowing pharmaceutical companies to maintain cultures of secrecy that prioritize corporate interests over patient safety.

The Path to Real Oversight

Transforming pharmaceutical inspection from theater to meaningful oversight will require fundamental changes in regulatory authority, inspection practices, and enforcement mechanisms.

Unannounced Inspections

Meaningful pharmaceutical oversight requires the authority to conduct unannounced inspections that observe actual operating conditions rather than carefully prepared presentations. This change would require international agreements that give regulatory authorities greater access to foreign facilities.

Independent Monitoring

Long-term monitoring of pharmaceutical facilities should be conducted by independent third parties rather than company employees or government inspectors with limited resources. These monitors could provide real-time oversight of manufacturing operations and quality control processes.

Enhanced Enforcement Authority

Regulatory agencies need enhanced authority to immediately halt operations at facilities with serious safety problems, rather than relying on slow bureaucratic processes that allow contaminated medications to continue reaching patients.

Whistleblower Protection

Strengthened legal protections for pharmaceutical industry whistleblowers could provide regulatory authorities with critical information about safety problems that would otherwise remain hidden within corporate structures.

The COVID-19 Inspection Collapse

The COVID-19 pandemic exposed the fragility of pharmaceutical inspection systems when travel restrictions and health concerns effectively shut down international oversight for months. During this period, millions of patients continued taking medications manufactured in facilities that received no regulatory oversight whatsoever.

The Virtual Inspection Experiment

Faced with the inability to conduct in-person inspections, the FDA attempted to implement "virtual inspections" conducted through video calls and document sharing. These remote inspections revealed just how much the traditional inspection process depends on physical presence and direct observation.

Virtual inspections allowed facility managers even greater control over what inspectors could see and evaluate. Companies could carefully stage video tours, control camera angles to avoid problematic areas, and present pre-selected documentation without allowing inspectors to request additional materials or explore concerning findings.

The limitations of virtual inspections became apparent when several contamination events occurred at facilities that had recently passed remote inspections, demonstrating that virtual oversight provides even less protection than traditional in-person visits.

The Backlog Crisis

As travel restrictions lifted, the FDA faced a massive backlog of overdue inspections at both domestic and international facilities. Some facilities that were supposed to be inspected annually hadn't been visited in over two years, creating gaps in oversight that allowed quality problems to persist undetected.

The agency's attempts to address this backlog by conducting shorter, more focused inspections further reduced the likelihood of detecting sophisticated quality problems or systematic safety issues. Facilities that might have been struggling with contamination or quality control failures for months received abbreviated inspections that were unlikely to identify these problems.

The Staffing Shortage Reality

The pandemic also highlighted the FDA's chronic understaffing of inspection operations. When several experienced inspectors left the agency during the pandemic, their expertise was not quickly replaced, further reducing the already limited oversight capacity.

New inspectors require extensive training to understand pharmaceutical manufacturing processes and identify potential safety problems. The loss of experienced staff during the pandemic created knowledge gaps that may take years to address, during which time inspection quality and effectiveness are compromised.

The Corporate Capture of Inspection Standards

The pharmaceutical industry's influence over inspection practices extends beyond individual facility visits to include the development of inspection standards and protocols that govern how oversight is conducted.

Industry Input on Inspection Guidelines

Pharmaceutical trade associations regularly provide input on FDA inspection guidelines, effectively allowing the industry to help write the rules by which they'll be evaluated. This input process creates opportunities for companies to shape inspection standards in ways that minimize the likelihood of discovering quality problems.

Industry representatives often argue that certain inspection practices are "impractical" or "disruptive" to manufacturing operations, leading to modifications in inspection protocols that reduce their effectiveness in identifying safety issues.

The Harmonization Trap

International efforts to "harmonize" pharmaceutical inspection standards often result in adopting the lowest common denominator approaches rather than the most protective practices. These harmonization efforts are typically driven by industry desires to reduce regulatory compliance costs rather than patient safety considerations.

When inspection standards are harmonized internationally, countries with more rigorous oversight practices may be pressured to adopt less stringent approaches to maintain consistency with international partners who prioritize industry convenience over patient protection.

The Self-Assessment Expansion

Increasingly, regulatory agencies are allowing pharmaceutical companies to conduct "self-assessments" and internal audits that substitute for traditional government inspections. These self-assessment programs allow companies to evaluate their own compliance while providing regulators with documentation that creates an appearance of oversight.

The obvious conflict of interest in allowing companies to inspect themselves is justified by claims that industry has better technical expertise and more detailed knowledge of their operations than government inspectors. However, these programs essentially ask companies to police themselves and report their own violations, creating obvious incentives for minimizing or concealing problems.

The Data Manipulation Epidemic

Modern pharmaceutical manufacturing generates vast amounts of electronic data that can be easily manipulated to conceal quality problems from inspectors, creating a new category of inspection challenges that traditional oversight methods are poorly equipped to address.

The Electronic Trail Deception

Sophisticated pharmaceutical companies have learned to manipulate electronic manufacturing and testing data in ways that are difficult for inspectors to detect. These manipulations can include:

Selective deletion of failed test results while retaining passing results

Retroactive modification of batch production records to eliminate evidence of deviations

Use of multiple computer systems to segregate problematic data from routine inspection reviews

Creation of parallel documentation systems that present sanitized versions of manufacturing activities

The Audit Trail Gaps

Many pharmaceutical facilities use computer systems that don't maintain complete audit trails of data modifications, making it impossible for inspectors to determine whether information has been altered or deleted. These systems may show current data status without revealing the history of changes that led to final results.

Facilities can exploit these audit trail gaps to present misleading information during inspections while technically maintaining electronic records that satisfy basic regulatory requirements.

The Forensic Analysis Shortage

FDA inspectors typically lack the forensic data analysis skills needed to detect sophisticated data manipulation or to identify patterns that might indicate systematic quality problems. This skills gap allows companies to present misleading information while confident that inspectors won't have the technical capability to uncover deception.

The agency's limited investment in training inspectors on advanced data analysis techniques means that sophisticated data manipulation schemes may never be detected, allowing facilities to maintain facades of compliance while actually operating with significant quality problems.

The International Standards Arbitrage

Pharmaceutical companies often exploit differences in international inspection standards by shifting problematic operations to countries with less rigorous oversight while maintaining compliant operations in countries with more stringent requirements.

The Regulatory Shopping Strategy

Companies may choose manufacturing locations based on regulatory convenience rather than operational efficiency, concentrating risky or cost-sensitive operations in countries with limited inspection resources or less stringent enforcement practices.

This regulatory arbitrage allows companies to benefit from weak oversight in some locations while maintaining reputations for quality based on their operations in more tightly regulated markets.

The Standards Export Problem

When pharmaceutical companies operate facilities in multiple countries, they may implement different quality standards depending on local regulatory requirements rather than maintaining consistent global standards based on best practices.

Facilities producing medications for American patients may operate under different quality standards than those producing for European markets, creating situations where American patients receive medications manufactured under less stringent oversight than patients in other countries.

The inspection game currently being played in pharmaceutical manufacturing prioritizes the appearance of oversight over actual patient protection. Until we acknowledge that the current system serves industry interests rather than public health, and until we implement reforms that provide meaningful regulatory oversight, patients will continue to be exposed to preventable risks from medications that should be healing rather than harming them.

The next time you hear that a medication is "FDA approved" or that manufacturing facilities are "regularly inspected," remember that these assurances may be based more on paperwork and theater than on actual verification of safety and quality. Real pharmaceutical oversight requires fundamental reforms that prioritize patient protection over industry convenience, but we're nowhere near that goal yet.

Chapter 9: Recalls You Never Heard About

I first realized how broken the pharmaceutical recall system was when I discovered that one of pituitary medications had been recalled six months earlier—and nobody had bothered to tell me. Not my doctor, not my pharmacist, not my insurance company. I only found out by accident while researching contamination issues for this book, when I stumbled across an obscure FDA database listing that mentioned my specific medication and lot numbers.

The recall notice was buried in technical language on a government website that most patients would never think to check. It mentioned "potential contamination with trace amounts of a probable carcinogen" but provided no information about health risks, no guidance for patients who had been taking the recalled medication, and no clear instructions about what actions to take.

When I called my doctor's office, they had no record of the recall. When I contacted my pharmacist, they claimed they had sent out notifications, though I had never received any. When I called the pharmaceutical company directly, they referred me back to the FDA website and declined to provide any additional information about potential health risks.

This experience taught me that the pharmaceutical recall system is designed to protect companies and regulatory agencies rather than patients. Recalls are conducted in ways that minimize public attention, legal liability, and regulatory embarrassment while leaving patients unknowingly exposed to dangerous medications for months or years after safety problems are identified.

The Hidden Recall Universe

Most patients assume that when medications are recalled for safety reasons, they'll be promptly notified and given clear guidance about protecting their health. The reality is that the vast majority of pharmaceutical recalls receive no public attention whatsoever, and patients who have consumed recalled medications are often never informed about potential risks.

The Classification Shell Game

The FDA classifies drug recalls into three categories that determine how much attention they receive and what actions are required to protect patients:

Class I recalls involve products that could cause serious health problems or death. These recalls typically receive some media attention and may trigger direct patient notification efforts.

Class II recalls involve products that might cause temporary health problems or pose only a slight threat of serious adverse effects. These recalls receive minimal public attention and limited patient notification.

Class III recalls involve products that are unlikely to cause adverse health effects but violate FDA regulations in some way. These recalls are essentially invisible to the public and patients.

The classification system allows pharmaceutical companies and regulators to minimize the apparent significance of most recalls by categorizing obviously dangerous situations as Class II or III rather than Class I. A medication contaminated with cancer-causing chemicals might be classified as Class II if the contamination levels are deemed "unlikely" to cause immediate harm, even though long-term health risks could be substantial.

The Voluntary Recall Deception

The vast majority of pharmaceutical recalls are classified as "voluntary," meaning that companies agree to remove products from the market in cooperation with the FDA rather than under direct regulatory order. This voluntary classification suggests that companies are proactively protecting patient safety when they're actually responding to regulatory pressure or public exposure of safety problems.

Voluntary recalls allow companies to control the timing, scope, and messaging around product removals in ways that minimize negative publicity and legal liability. Companies can delay recall announcements until favorable news cycles, limit recalls to specific batches while continuing to sell other potentially problematic products, and frame recall communications to minimize apparent safety risks.

The Retail Level Deception

Many pharmaceutical recalls are classified as "retail level" recalls, meaning that products are removed from pharmacy shelves but patients who have already purchased the medications are not directly notified. This classification allows companies and regulators to claim they've addressed safety problems while leaving patients unknowingly consuming dangerous medications.

Retail level recalls are particularly problematic for medications that patients take regularly over extended periods. A patient might continue taking a recalled blood pressure medication for months after it's been removed from pharmacy shelves, never knowing that the medication has been deemed unsafe for consumption.

The Patient Notification Failure

When pharmaceutical recalls do attempt to notify patients, the communication systems used are often inadequate, confusing, or designed more to limit legal liability than to protect patient health.

The Lot Number Labyrinth

Most recall notifications require patients to check specific lot numbers printed in small text on medication packaging to determine whether their products are affected. This system assumes that patients retain medication packaging, can locate tiny lot numbers on bottles and boxes, and understand how to interpret complex alphanumeric codes.

Many patients discard medication packaging immediately, making it impossible to determine whether their medications are subject to recalls. Others may be able to locate lot numbers but find the recall notifications too technical or confusing to understand whether they're affected.

The lot number system also fails patients who take multiple medications from the same manufacturer, as they may need to check dozens of various products against lengthy lists of recalled lot numbers without clear guidance about prioritization or risk levels.

The Healthcare Provider Gap

Recall notifications often assume that healthcare providers will inform their patients about recalled medications, but most doctors and pharmacists lack systems for tracking which specific products their patients are taking or for efficiently communicating recall information.

Electronic health records typically track medications by name and dose rather than specific lot numbers or manufacturers, making it difficult for healthcare providers to identify patients who might be affected by specific recalls. Even when providers can identify affected patients, they may lack current contact information or efficient communication systems for reaching patients quickly.

The Language and Literacy Barriers

Recall notifications are typically written in technical language that assumes patients understand pharmaceutical terminology, regulatory processes, and health risk assessment. These communications often fail to clearly explain what actions patients should take or how to assess their personal risk from recalled medications.

Patients with limited English proficiency, low health literacy, or cognitive impairments may be unable to understand recall notifications even when they receive them. The complex, legalistic language used in most recall communications seems designed more to limit legal liability than to ensure patient comprehension.

The Timing Manipulation

Pharmaceutical companies and regulatory agencies routinely manipulate the timing of recall announcements to minimize media attention and public concern, often delaying announcements until news cycles are dominated by other events or scheduling releases for times when public attention is elsewhere.

The Friday Night News Dump

Many pharmaceutical recalls are announced on Friday evenings or before holiday weekends, when media attention is minimal and the public is least likely to notice. This timing manipulation allows companies to claim they've fulfilled their notification obligations while ensuring that most patients never learn about the recalls.

The Friday night news dump strategy is particularly common for recalls involving medications taken by large numbers of patients or products that might generate significant public concern. By timing announcements strategically, companies can often ensure that recall news disappears from public attention before most patients become aware of the safety issues.

The Competitive Event Timing

Recall announcements are sometimes delayed or accelerated to coincide with major news events that will dominate media coverage. Companies may delay recall announcements until public attention is focused on political crises, natural disasters, or other major stories that will overshadow pharmaceutical safety news.

This competitive event timing allows companies to minimize the reputational and fiscal impact of recalls while technically complying with regulatory requirements for public notification.

The Gradual Disclosure Strategy

Some companies manage recall timing by gradually disclosing safety information over extended periods rather than announcing comprehensive recalls all at once. This strategy allows companies to minimize the apparent scope of safety problems while controlling the pace of public disclosure.

A company might initially announce a limited recall affecting specific lot numbers, then gradually expand the recall scope over weeks or months as additional safety information becomes available. This gradual disclosure prevents the concentrated media attention that might result from announcing a comprehensive recall involving millions of medication doses.

The Scope Limitation Game

Pharmaceutical companies often limit the scope of recalls to minimize their apparent significance and reduce legal liability, even when safety problems may affect broader product ranges or patient populations.

The Batch Segmentation Strategy

Companies frequently limit recalls to specific manufacturing batches even when safety problems may be systemic issues affecting multiple production runs. This batch segmentation allows companies to characterize widespread quality problems as isolated manufacturing errors.

A contamination problem that affects an entire manufacturing facility might be addressed through a series of small batch recalls rather than a comprehensive facility recalls, minimizing the apparent scope of the safety issue while potentially leaving other contaminated products on the market.

The Geographic Limitation Tactic

Some recalls are limited to specific geographic regions even when safety problems may affect products distributed more widely. Companies might recall products from markets where regulatory pressure is strongest while continuing to sell potentially dangerous products in areas with less regulatory oversight.

This geographic limitation allows companies to respond to immediate regulatory pressure while maintaining revenue from unaffected markets, even when the underlying safety problems may affect all products from the same manufacturing processes.

The Indication-Specific Recall

Companies sometimes limit recalls to medications approved for specific medical conditions while continuing to sell identical products approved for different uses. This indication-specific approach allows companies to minimize recall scope while potentially leaving patients with other conditions exposed to the same safety risks.

A medication might be recalled for use in treating high blood pressure while remaining available for treating heart rhythm disorders, even though the safety problem affects the medication regardless of its prescribed use.

The Post-Recall Abandonment

Perhaps the most troubling aspect of pharmaceutical recalls is the complete abandonment of patients after recall announcements are made. Companies and regulatory agencies typically provide no follow-up support, health monitoring, or guidance for patients who may have been harmed by recalled medications.

The Health Monitoring Void

When medications are recalled for safety reasons, patients who have been taking these products are rarely offered health monitoring or screening to detect potential adverse effects. This monitoring void means that health problems caused by recalled medications may go undetected or be attributed to other causes.

Patients who consumed NDMA-contaminated blood pressure medications for years before recalls were announced have received no systematic cancer screening or health monitoring, despite evidence that NDMA exposure increases cancer risk. These patients are left to wonder whether their medication exposure will affect their long-term health while receiving no medical support for addressing their concerns.

The Treatment Transition Crisis

Patients taking recalled medications often face difficulties obtaining alternative treatments, particularly when recalls affect multiple products or entire medication classes. Healthcare providers may be unprepared to manage sudden treatment transitions for large numbers of patients simultaneously.

The treatment transition crisis is particularly problematic for patients taking medications for chronic conditions that require stable therapeutic levels. Sudden switches to alternative medications can destabilize patients' health while they adjust to different formulations, dosing schedules, or side effect profiles.

The Legal Limbo Problem

Patients who believe they've been harmed by recalled medications often find themselves in legal limbo, unable to obtain clear information about their rights or access to compensation. Pharmaceutical companies typically deny liability for recalled products while regulatory agencies disclaim responsibility for individual patient outcomes.

This legal limbo leaves patients bearing the financial and health consequences of pharmaceutical company negligence while being unable to obtain adequate legal recourse or medical support for addressing potential harm.

The Recall Communication Blackout

The systems used to communicate recall information to patients are so inadequate that most recalls remain essentially invisible to the people they're supposed to protect.

The Website Burial Strategy

Most recall information is published only on obscure government websites that patients would never think to check. The FDA's recall database is difficult to navigate, uses technical language that most patients can't understand, and provides no painless way for patients to determine whether medications they're taking are subject to recalls.

Pharmaceutical companies typically publish recall information only on their corporate websites, often in sections devoted to regulatory compliance rather than patient safety. These corporate recall notices are written in legal language designed to limit liability rather than inform patients about health risks.

The Media Dependence Problem

Patients typically learn about pharmaceutical recalls only when major media outlets choose to cover specific cases, but most recalls receive no media attention whatsoever. This media dependence means that patient awareness of recalls depends more on journalistic judgment about newsworthiness than on actual health risks.

The media's focus on dramatic or unusual recall cases means that patients may be well-informed about rare, high-profile recalls while remaining completely unaware of more common recalls that might actually affect their medications.

The Healthcare Provider Information Gap

Healthcare providers often know little more than patients about ongoing recalls, as they typically receive recall information through the same inadequate channels available to the general public. Medical offices and pharmacies may not have systems for actively monitoring recall databases or efficiently communicating recall information to affected patients.

This healthcare provider information gap means that patients can't rely on their doctors or pharmacists to inform them about recalls affecting their medications, leaving them dependent on their own research and vigilance to identify potential safety issues.

The International Recall Disparities

The adequacy of pharmaceutical recall systems varies dramatically between countries, revealing how arbitrary and inadequate American recall practices are compared to more protective international approaches.

The European Transparency Advantage

European pharmaceutical recall systems typically provide much more comprehensive patient notification and clearer information about health risks than American systems. European recalls often include direct patient notification requirements, clearer risk communication, and more comprehensive product removal from the marketplace.

European regulatory agencies also maintain more accessible recall databases with better search capabilities and clearer explanations of health risks in multiple languages. These systems make it much easier for patients to determine whether their medications are subject to recalls and what actions they should take to protect their health.

The Canadian Communication Standards

Canadian pharmaceutical recalls typically include more detailed patient communication requirements and clearer guidance about alternative treatments. Canadian recalls often provide specific recommendations for healthcare providers about managing patient transitions to alternative medications.

The Canadian recall system also includes more comprehensive follow-up requirements that ensure recalled products are actually removed from the marketplace and that patients receive adequate support during treatment transitions.

The Regulatory Race to the Bottom

Despite evidence that other countries provide better recall protection for patients, American pharmaceutical companies often lobby against adopting more protective international practices, arguing that enhanced recall requirements would be burdensome and costly to implement.

This resistance to international best practices means that American patients receive less protection from pharmaceutical recalls than patients in many other developed countries, despite Americans often paying higher prices for the same medications.

The Digital Age Recall Failure

Modern technology could dramatically improve pharmaceutical recall communication and patient protection, but companies and regulatory agencies have made minimal investments in developing effective digital notification systems.

The Social Media Silence

Pharmaceutical companies maintain extensive social media presences for marketing their products but rarely use these platforms to communicate recall information to patients. Companies that spend millions on social media advertising often provide no recall notifications through the same channels.

This social media silence means that patients who might be highly engaged with pharmaceutical companies' marketing communications receive no recall information through the digital platforms they use most frequently.

The Mobile Technology Gap

Despite widespread smartphone adoption, very few pharmaceutical recall systems take advantage of mobile technology to reach patients quickly and effectively. Mobile apps could provide immediate recall notifications to patients taking specific medications, but such systems remain rare and underdeveloped.

The mobile technology gap represents a missed opportunity to dramatically improve recall communication effectiveness, particularly for younger patients who rely primarily on mobile devices for information and communication.

The Electronic Health Record Integration Failure

Electronic health record systems could automatically identify patients taking recalled medications and trigger notification systems, but most healthcare providers lack the technical infrastructure or procedures to implement such systems effectively.

This integration failure means that electronic health records, which contain detailed information about patients' medication use, remain disconnected from recall notification systems that could protect patient safety.

The Path to Recall Reform

Transforming pharmaceutical recalls from industry protection mechanisms to patient safety systems will require fundamental changes in notification requirements, communication standards, and accountability measures.

Mandatory Direct Notification

All pharmaceutical recalls should require direct notification to patients through multiple communication channels, including mail, email, text messages, and phone calls. These notifications should be written in plain language that clearly explains health risks and necessary actions.

Real-Time Digital Integration

Recall information should be automatically integrated into electronic health records, pharmacy databases, and mobile health applications to ensure that patients and healthcare providers receive immediate notification when medications they're taking are recalled.

Enhanced Accountability Measures

Companies that fail to adequately notify patients about recalls should face significant financial penalties and increased regulatory oversight. Current systems that allow companies to hide recalls behind technical language and obscure websites should be replaced with requirements for prominent, clear public notification.

Comprehensive Health Monitoring

Patients who have consumed recalled medications should be offered systematic health monitoring and screening to detect potential adverse effects. This monitoring should be funded by the pharmaceutical companies responsible for the safety problems rather than by patients or healthcare systems.

The pharmaceutical recall system represents one of the most glaring failures in American healthcare's approach to patient safety. Millions of patients continue taking dangerous medications long after safety problems have been identified, not because the problems can't be addressed, but because the recall system is designed to protect industry interests rather than patient health.

Until we acknowledge that pharmaceutical recalls should prioritize patient protection over corporate liability management, and until we implement systems that ensure patients are promptly and clearly informed about medication safety issues, patients will continue to serve as unknowing victims of a recall system that treats their health as less important than pharmaceutical industry profits.

The next time you hear about a pharmaceutical recall, remember that for every recall that makes the news, dozens of others remain hidden in obscure databases and technical communications that most patients will never see. Your safety depends not on a functioning recall system, but on your own vigilance in monitoring for problems that companies and regulators may never tell you about.

Chapter 10: Over-the-Counter Dangers

The discovery that changed everything for me wasn't in a prescription medication—it was in a simple over-the-counter sinus medication I'd been taking for seasonal allergies. After my experience with hidden soy and dairy in prescription drugs, I had become obsessive about reading ingredient labels on everything I consumed. When I picked up my usual sinus medication at the pharmacy, I decided to scrutinize the fine print on the package.

Buried in the inactive ingredient list, in tiny text that required reading glasses to decipher, I found it: soy lecithin. The same allergen that had been causing my digestive problems was hiding in what I thought was a simple, harmless allergy medication. But this was just the beginning of what would become a months-long investigation into the hidden chemical reality of over-the-counter medications.

What I discovered shocked me more than anything I'd learned about prescription drugs. Over-the-counter medications—the products we trust enough to buy without prescriptions, give to our children, and take without consulting doctors—are often more contaminated with unnecessary chemicals than prescription medications. They contain higher levels of artificial dyes, more preservatives, more allergens, and more industrial chemicals than many prescription drugs, yet they receive far less regulatory oversight and far less public scrutiny.

The over-the-counter drug industry has convinced millions of Americans that "non-prescription" means "safe," when in reality it often means "less regulated, less monitored, and more chemically complex." These medications represent a massive uncontrolled experiment in chemical exposure that affects virtually every American, from infants taking liquid pain relievers to elderly patients managing chronic conditions with daily OTC regimens.

The False Security of "Non-Prescription"

The pharmaceutical industry has masterfully exploited the public's assumption that over-the-counter medications are inherently safer than prescription drugs. This assumption allows OTC manufacturers to include chemical additives and use manufacturing practices that would trigger scrutiny if used in prescription medications.

The Regulatory Double Standard

Over-the-counter medications are subject to significantly less stringent regulatory oversight than prescription drugs. While prescription medications require extensive clinical trials and detailed safety documentation, OTC drugs often gain approval through "monograph" systems that group similar ingredients together and assume safety based on historical use rather than rigorous testing.

This regulatory double standard means that OTC medications can include untested combinations of ingredients, use higher levels of potentially dangerous additives, and employ manufacturing processes that wouldn't be acceptable for prescription drugs. The result is a category of medications that many people take daily without realizing they may be more chemically hazardous than the prescription drugs they're trying to avoid.

The Self-Medication Delusion

The marketing of OTC medications encourages a dangerous self-medication culture that treats these products as harmless consumer goods rather than potent chemical compounds. Advertisements for OTC drugs focus on convenience and immediate relief while minimizing discussion of chemical ingredients, potential side effects, or long-term health consequences.

This marketing approach encourages people to take OTC medications more frequently, in higher doses, and for longer periods than would be appropriate for prescription drugs with similar chemical profiles. The result is often higher cumulative chemical exposure from OTC medications than from prescription drugs that receive much more careful medical supervision.

The Combination Product Nightmare

Many OTC medications contain multiple active ingredients combined with extensive lists of inactive chemicals, creating complex chemical mixtures that have never been tested for safety as complete formulations. A typical cold medication might contain pain relievers, decongestants, antihistamines, expectorants, and dozens of inactive ingredients, yet the safety of this chemical cocktail has never been systematically evaluated.

These combination products often expose consumers to active ingredients they don't need while delivering unnecessarily high chemical loads through extensive inactive ingredient lists. Someone taking an OTC cold medication for congestion might also be consuming pain relievers, artificial stimulants, and preservatives they don't need and that could cause adverse effects or interact with other medications.

The Soy Contamination Web

My discovery of soy lecithin in sinus medications led me down a research rabbit hole that revealed the extent to which soy derivatives contaminate the OTC medication supply. Soy appears in over-the-counter drugs in dozens of different forms, often disguised under chemical names that give no indication of their agricultural origins.

Hidden Soy in Common OTC Medications

Sinus and Allergy Medications: Nearly every major brand of sinus medication contains soy lecithin as an emulsifier or binding agent. Claritin, Sudafed, Benadryl, and dozens of generic equivalents all contain soy derivatives that can trigger reactions in sensitive individuals.

Cough Medicines: Liquid cough medications are particularly problematic for soy-sensitive individuals because they often contain multiple soy derivatives. Robitussin, Delsym, and most store-brand cough syrups contain soy lecithin, soy protein isolates, or other soy-derived emulsifiers that help maintain the medication's consistency and shelf stability.

Pain Relievers: Many over-the-counter pain medications contain soy-derived lubricants and binding agents. Even seemingly simple products like generic ibuprofen or acetaminophen tablets often contain soy lecithin or other soy derivatives that serve manufacturing functions.

Digestive Medications: The irony is particularly cruel with digestive medications—products designed to treat stomach problems often contain soy derivatives that can cause digestive symptoms in sensitive individuals. Antacids, anti-diarrheal medications, and stomach acid reducers frequently contain soy lecithin as a texture modifier.

The Chemical Name Disguise

Soy derivatives appear in OTC medications under numerous chemical names that obscure their agricultural origins:

Lecithin: Usually derived from soybeans unless specifically labeled otherwise

Polysorbate 80: Often manufactured using soy-derived fatty acids

Vitamin E (tocopherols): Frequently extracted from soybean oil

Monoglycerides and diglycerides: Often derived from soy oil

Sodium stearoyl lactylate: May be produced using soy-derived stearic acid

This chemical name disguise makes it nearly impossible for soy-sensitive individuals to identify problematic products without conducting extensive research into manufacturing processes and ingredient sourcing.

The Cross-Contamination Reality

Even OTC medications that don't intentionally contain soy ingredients may be contaminated through shared manufacturing equipment or facilities. Many pharmaceutical manufacturers produce both soy-containing and soy-free products using the same equipment, creating opportunities for cross-contamination that can trigger reactions in overly sensitive individuals.

This cross-contamination problem is particularly acute in facilities that produce both food products and pharmaceuticals, as soy is ubiquitous in processed food manufacturing and can contaminate pharmaceutical production lines through shared equipment or airborne particles.

The Pediatric Chemical Assault

Children's over-the-counter medications represent perhaps the most egregious example of unnecessary chemical exposure in the pharmaceutical industry. These products are specifically formulated to appeal to children through bright colors, sweet flavors, and candy-like appearances, often containing higher concentrations of artificial additives than adult formulations.

The Flavor and Color Overload

Children's OTC medications typically contain extensive artificial flavoring and coloring systems designed to make medicine-taking a pleasant experience rather than a medical necessity. These flavoring systems often include:

Multiple artificial sweeteners: Aspartame, sucralose, and saccharin are commonly combined to create appealing taste profiles

Petroleum-derived dyes: Red 40, Yellow 6, and Blue 1 are routinely used to create visually appealing medications

Synthetic flavoring compounds: Dozens of artificial chemicals are combined to create "grape," "cherry," or "bubble gum" flavors that bear no resemblance to natural flavors

The Dosing Multiplication Problem

Children's medications are often administered multiple times per day over extended periods, multiplying their exposure to artificial additives far beyond what would occur with occasional adult use. A child taking liquid pain reliever four times daily for a week might consume more artificial dyes and preservatives than an adult taking prescription medications for months.

This dosing multiplication is particularly problematic for artificial dyes and preservatives that have been linked to behavioral problems in children. The very medications being used to treat children's illnesses may be contributing to attention problems, hyperactivity, and other behavioral issues through their extensive artificial additive content.

The Infant Formula Connection

Many infant medications contain ingredients similar to those found in infant formula, but in much higher concentrations and with additional preservatives and stabilizers. Infant Tylenol, for example, contains artificial sweeteners and preservatives that wouldn't be acceptable in infant formula but are somehow considered appropriate for sick babies.

The logic of including artificial sweeteners in infant medications is particularly questionable, as babies haven't yet developed preferences for sweet tastes and don't require flavor enhancement to accept necessary medications.

The Acetaminophen Epidemic

Acetaminophen, the active ingredient in Tylenol and hundreds of other OTC medications, represents one of the most dangerous substances routinely available without prescription. Despite being responsible for more emergency room visits and liver failures than any other medication, acetaminophen continues to be marketed as a safe, family-friendly pain reliever.

The Liver Destruction Reality

Acetaminophen is directly toxic to liver cells, and the margin between therapeutic doses and liver-damaging doses is smaller than most people realize. The maximum recommended daily dose of acetaminophen (4,000 milligrams) can cause liver damage in some individuals, particularly those who consume alcohol, have pre-existing liver problems, or take other medications that affect liver function.

The over-the-counter availability of acetaminophen has created a false sense of security that leads to widespread overdosing and dangerous drug interactions. Many people take multiple acetaminophen-containing products simultaneously without realizing they're exceeding safe dosage limits.

The Hidden Acetaminophen Problem

Acetaminophen appears in dozens of OTC combination products where consumers might not realize they're consuming this liver-toxic ingredient. Cold medications, sinus treatments, sleep aids, and even some allergy medications contain acetaminophen combined with other active ingredients.

This hidden acetaminophen creates opportunities for accidental overdoses when people take multiple OTC products containing the ingredient. Someone taking Tylenol for pain while also using NyQuil for cold symptoms might unknowingly consume dangerous levels of acetaminophen.

The Alcohol Interaction Crisis

The combination of acetaminophen and alcohol creates particularly dangerous liver toxicity risks that are poorly understood by most consumers. Even moderate alcohol consumption can dramatically increase acetaminophen's liver-damaging potential, yet this interaction is minimally communicated in OTC marketing and labeling.

Many people routinely combine acetaminophen use with social drinking without realizing they're creating conditions for serious liver damage. The casual marketing of acetaminophen as a hangover remedy is particularly irresponsible given the dangerous interaction between alcohol and this medication.

The Antihistamine Dependence Cycle

Over-the-counter antihistamines, marketed for allergies and sleep problems, often create psychological and physiological dependencies that trap consumers in cycles of increasing use and decreasing effectiveness.

The Tolerance Development

Regular use of OTC antihistamines often leads to tolerance, where consumers need higher doses or more frequent administration to achieve the same effects. This tolerance development can lead to chronic overuse of these medications and exposure to unnecessary chemical loads.

The tolerance problem is particularly acute with sleep aids containing diphenhydramine (Benadryl), where consumers often escalate doses far beyond recommended levels in attempts to maintain sleep-promoting effects.

The Rebound Effect

Discontinuing regular antihistamine use often triggers rebound effects where allergy symptoms or sleep problems become worse than they were before medication use began. These rebound effects can trap consumers in cycles of increasing medication dependence.

The rebound effect is poorly understood by most consumers, who interpret worsening symptoms as evidence that they need to continue or increase their medication use rather than recognizing that the medications themselves may be contributing to their problems.

The Cognitive Impact

Regular antihistamine use, particularly of older compounds like diphenhydramine, can cause significant cognitive impairment including memory problems, confusion, and decreased mental sharpness. These cognitive effects are often attributed to allergies or sleep problems rather than recognized as medication side effects.

Long-term antihistamine use has been linked to increased dementia risk in elderly patients, yet these medications continue to be marketed for daily use in managing chronic allergy symptoms.

The Supplement-Medication Boundary Blur

The line between over-the-counter medications and dietary supplements has become increasingly blurred, creating regulatory gaps that allow products with drug-like effects to avoid pharmaceutical oversight while exposing consumers to unpredictable chemical mixtures.

The Regulatory Arbitrage

Many products that function as medications are marketed as dietary supplements to avoid FDA drug regulation. These products often contain potent bioactive compounds that can cause significant physiological effects and drug interactions, yet they're subject to minimal safety oversight.

Sleep aids, weight loss products, and energy supplements often contain pharmaceutical-grade compounds that would require prescription oversight if marketed as medications but avoid regulation by claiming to be nutritional supplements.

The Manufacturing Quality Gap

Supplement manufacturing facilities are subject to much less stringent quality control requirements than pharmaceutical facilities, creating opportunities for contamination, mislabeling, and quality problems that would be unacceptable in OTC drug manufacturing.

Many supplements contain pharmaceutical ingredients at unpredictable concentrations, creating risks of overdose or underdose that consumers can't anticipate. The lack of standardized manufacturing processes means that identical products from the same manufacturer might contain dramatically different ingredient levels.

The Drug Interaction Risks

Supplements often contain multiple bioactive compounds that can interact with prescription medications in dangerous ways, yet healthcare providers typically receive minimal information about supplement ingredients and potential interactions.

Consumers taking both OTC medications and supplements may be unknowingly creating dangerous drug interactions through combinations that have never been tested for safety.

The Foreign Manufacturing Free-for-All

Over-the-counter medications are increasingly manufactured in overseas facilities with minimal quality control oversight, creating risks of contamination and quality problems that can affect millions of consumers before problems are detected.

The China Manufacturing Dominance

A significant percentage of OTC medications sold in America are manufactured in Chinese facilities that receive infrequent inspections and operate under quality standards that differ from American requirements. These facilities often produce medications for multiple global markets using different quality standards depending on destination countries.

The concentration of OTC manufacturing in China creates supply chain vulnerabilities that became apparent during COVID-19 pandemic disruptions, when shortages of basic OTC medications revealed the extent of American dependence on foreign manufacturing.

The Quality Control Arbitrage

OTC manufacturers often choose manufacturing locations based on cost considerations rather than quality standards, concentrating production in countries with minimal regulatory oversight and enforcement.

This quality control arbitrage allows companies to reduce manufacturing costs while potentially exposing American consumers to products that wouldn't meet domestic quality standards.

The Inspection Gap

Foreign facilities manufacturing OTC medications receive even less regulatory oversight than facilities producing prescription drugs, as OTC products are considered lower priority for international inspection efforts.

Many facilities producing popular OTC brands have never been inspected by American regulators, despite supplying medications consumed by millions of Americans daily.

The Marketing Deception Matrix

The marketing of over-the-counter medications relies on deceptive practices that minimize chemical risks while maximizing perceived safety and effectiveness.

The "Natural" Ingredient Myth

Many OTC medications claim to contain "natural" ingredients while actually including synthetic versions of naturally occurring compounds or natural ingredients that have been chemically modified through industrial processes.

These "natural" marketing claims create false impressions of safety while obscuring the extensive chemical processing and artificial additives used in OTC formulations.

The "Doctor Recommended" Manipulation

OTC marketing frequently claims that products are "doctor recommended" or "pharmacist preferred" based on limited surveys or promotional programs rather than comprehensive medical evaluations.

These endorsement claims create false impressions of medical approval while failing to disclose potential conflicts of interest or the limited scope of professional recommendations.

The Symptom Multiplication Strategy

OTC marketing often encourages consumers to treat normal physiological processes as medical conditions requiring chemical intervention. Seasonal allergies, occasional sleeplessness, and minor digestive upset are presented as serious conditions requiring daily medication.

This symptom multiplication creates markets for chronic OTC medication use that expose consumers to unnecessary chemical loads while generating profits for pharmaceutical companies.

The Elderly Vulnerability Crisis

Elderly consumers are particularly vulnerable to OTC medication risks due to age-related changes in drug metabolism, increased likelihood of drug interactions, and marketing that specifically targets older adults with chronic health concerns.

The Polypharmacy Amplification

Elderly consumers often take multiple OTC medications simultaneously, creating complex chemical exposures that have never been tested for safety in combination. The addition of OTC medications to prescription drug regimens can create dangerous interactions and cumulative toxicity.

The Cognitive Impairment Risk

Many OTC medications can cause or worsen cognitive impairment in elderly users, particularly antihistamines and sleep aids. These cognitive effects may be mistakenly attributed to aging or dementia rather than recognized as medication side effects.

The Marketing Targeting

OTC marketing specifically targets elderly consumers with messages about maintaining independence and managing chronic conditions, often encouraging inappropriate self-medication that should involve healthcare provider oversight.

The Path to OTC Reform

Reforming over-the-counter medication safety will require fundamental changes in regulatory oversight, manufacturing standards, and marketing practices.

Enhanced Regulatory Standards

OTC medications should be subject to the same safety testing and quality control requirements as prescription drugs, including comprehensive evaluation of inactive ingredients and combination product safety.

Improved Labeling Requirements

OTC medication labels should include clear, prominent disclosure of all chemical ingredients using plain language that consumers can understand, along with specific warnings about potential interactions and cumulative exposure risks.

Restricted Marketing Practices

Marketing of OTC medications should be subject to the same truth-in-advertising standards applied to prescription drugs, including requirements for balanced disclosure of risks and limitations on unsupported safety claims.

Manufacturing Oversight

Foreign facilities manufacturing OTC medications for American consumers should be subject to the same inspection and quality control requirements as domestic facilities, with mandatory quality certifications and regular oversight.

The over-the-counter medication system represents one of the largest uncontrolled experiments in chemical exposure affecting the American population. Millions of people consume these products daily without understanding their chemical complexity or potential health risks, trusting in a regulatory system that provides minimal oversight and a marketing system that prioritizes profits over safety.

My discovery of soy contamination in sinus medications opened my eyes to a world of hidden chemical exposure that affects virtually every American who uses OTC medications. Until we acknowledge that "non-prescription" doesn't mean "safe" and implement reforms that prioritize consumer protection over industry convenience, OTC medications will continue to represent a significant threat to public health disguised as consumer convenience.

The next time you reach for an over-the-counter medication, remember that you may be consuming a complex chemical mixture that has received less safety testing than the prescription drugs you're trying to avoid. Your health depends on understanding that OTC doesn't mean safe—it often means less regulated, less monitored, and potentially more dangerous than the prescription alternatives.

Chapter 11: The Money Trail

After months of researching pharmaceutical contamination, regulatory failures, and hidden chemical dangers, I kept returning to one fundamental question: Why does this system persist when it so obviously fails to protect patients? The answer, I discovered, lies in following the money. Every aspect of pharmaceutical manufacturing, regulation, and distribution is designed to maximize profits for industry stakeholders while minimizing costs—and patient safety has become just another cost to be minimized.

The pharmaceutical industry isn't accidentally exposing patients to dangerous chemicals while trying to help them. The contamination, the regulatory capture, the hidden ingredients, and the systematic concealment of safety information all exist because they're profitable. Companies make more money by cutting corners on safety than they would lose from lawsuits and regulatory penalties. The system isn't broken—it's working exactly as designed to enrich pharmaceutical companies at patients' expense.

What I found when I followed the money trail was a sophisticated network of financial incentives that reward companies for exposing patients to unnecessary risks while punishing those who prioritize safety over profits. This financial architecture explains why contamination problems persist for years before being addressed, why generic medications contain more dangerous chemicals than necessary, and why regulatory agencies consistently side with industry interests over patient protection.

The Cost-Cutting Imperative

The foundation of pharmaceutical industry profits rests on relentless cost reduction that treats patient safety as an obstacle to financial success rather than a fundamental responsibility.

Manufacturing to the Bottom Line

Every decision about pharmaceutical manufacturing is ultimately a financial calculation that weighs production costs against potential liability exposure. Companies routinely choose cheaper manufacturing processes, lower-quality raw materials, and less rigorous quality control systems because these choices increase short-term profits even when they increase long-term safety risks.

The move to overseas manufacturing wasn't driven by superior quality or better regulatory oversight—it was driven purely by labor cost savings and reduced environmental compliance costs. Companies discovered they could reduce manufacturing costs by 60-80% by moving production to countries with lower wages and less stringent safety regulations, while passing contamination and quality risks on to patients.

The Acceptable Risk Calculation

Pharmaceutical companies employ teams of actuaries and risk analysts who calculate the financial costs of safety problems and compare them to the costs of prevention. These calculations often conclude that paying settlements and regulatory fines is more profitable than implementing safety measures that would prevent contamination and quality problems.

Internal company documents obtained through litigation have revealed instances where companies discovered contamination problems but conducted cost-benefit analyses concluding that fixing the problems would be more expensive than managing the legal and regulatory consequences of continued contamination. In these calculations, patient health becomes just another line item in corporate profit optimization.

The Quality Control Trade-Off

Quality control represents a significant cost center for pharmaceutical manufacturers, and companies continuously seek ways to minimize these expenses while maintaining the appearance of adequate oversight. This has led to the widespread adoption of "risk-based" quality systems that reduce testing and oversight for products deemed "low risk"—often based on financial rather than safety considerations.

Companies may reduce quality control testing for medications with low profit margins while maintaining more rigorous oversight for high-revenue products. This approach means that cheaper medications often receive less safety oversight, exposing patients who can't afford expensive brand-name drugs to higher contamination and quality risks.

The Generic Gold Rush

The generic drug industry represents one of the most profitable segments of pharmaceutical manufacturing, built on a regulatory system that allows maximum cost-cutting with minimal safety oversight.

The Race to the Bottom

Generic drug pricing is primarily determined by manufacturing cost competition, creating powerful incentives for companies to reduce expenses through any means possible. This race to the bottom has led to the systematic degradation of manufacturing standards as companies compete to offer the lowest prices to pharmacy chains and insurance companies.

Generic manufacturers often win contracts by promising prices that are only achievable through extreme cost-cutting measures including the use of cheaper raw materials, reduced quality control testing, and manufacturing in facilities with minimal regulatory oversight. These cost reductions create safety risks that are passed on to patients while generating substantial profits for generic manufacturers.

The Volume Profit Model

Generic manufacturers compensate for low per-unit prices through massive production volumes, creating incentives to maximize manufacturing speed and minimize per-dose production costs. This volume-driven model encourages the use of automated production systems with minimal human oversight and quality control processes designed for speed rather than safety.

The pressure to maintain high production volumes can lead companies to continue manufacturing even when quality problems are identified, as production shutdowns represent significant financial losses. Companies may choose to recall products after they've been distributed rather than halt production when problems are discovered, exposing patients to contaminated medications while protecting manufacturing profits.

The Regulatory Arbitrage Advantage

Generic manufacturers have discovered they can maximize profits by exploiting differences in international regulatory standards, concentrating production in countries with the most permissive oversight while selling products in markets with higher prices. This regulatory arbitrage allows companies to benefit from reduced manufacturing costs while avoiding the safety compliance expenses required in more regulated markets.

Companies may operate the same facility under different quality standards depending on the destination markets for their products, producing lower-quality medications for cost-sensitive markets while maintaining higher standards for premium markets. This approach maximizes profits while exposing some patient populations to higher safety risks than others.

The Insurance Industry Enablers

Health insurance companies play a crucial role in perpetuating pharmaceutical safety problems by prioritizing cost savings over patient safety in their formulary decisions and coverage policies.

The Lowest-Price Mandate

Insurance companies routinely mandate the use of the cheapest available generic medications regardless of quality differences or patient-specific safety considerations. These lowest-price mandates create powerful market incentives for generic manufacturers to compete on cost rather than safety, driving the race to the bottom in manufacturing standards.

Patients who experience problems with mandated generic medications often find themselves trapped in insurance systems that refuse to cover safer alternatives even when medical necessity is documented. This creates a two-tiered system where medication safety depends on financial resources rather than medical need.

The Formulary Manipulation

Insurance company formularies—the lists of covered medications—are often designed based on financial kickbacks and rebate arrangements rather than medical effectiveness or safety considerations. Pharmaceutical companies pay substantial rebates to insurance companies in exchange for preferred formulary placement, creating conflicts of interest that prioritize cost savings over patient outcomes.

These formulary arrangements can force patients to use medications from manufacturers with poor safety records while blocking access to safer alternatives from companies that don't offer equivalent financial incentives to insurance companies.

The Prior Authorization Burden

Insurance companies use prior authorization requirements to discourage the use of more expensive medications even when safety considerations support their use. These administrative barriers often force patients and healthcare providers to accept cheaper alternatives rather than navigate complex approval processes for safer medications.

The prior authorization system creates financial incentives for healthcare providers to prescribe whatever medications receive automatic approval rather than spending time and resources advocating for optimal treatment choices. This system shifts medical decision-making from clinical considerations to administrative convenience.

The Regulatory Capture Economics

The relationship between pharmaceutical companies and regulatory agencies is fundamentally shaped by financial arrangements that create conflicts of interest favoring industry profits over patient protection.

The User Fee Dependency

The FDA's pharmaceutical oversight operations are largely funded through user fees paid by the pharmaceutical companies being regulated, creating an obvious conflict of interest where the agency depends financially on the industry it's supposed to police. This funding arrangement gives pharmaceutical companies significant leverage over regulatory decisions and creates pressure on the FDA to maintain positive relationships with industry.

The user fee system has grown to represent the majority of FDA's drug oversight budget, making the agency dependent on pharmaceutical industry payments for basic operations. This dependency relationship inevitably influences regulatory decisions in favor of industry interests when conflicts arise between company profits and patient safety.

The Revolving Door Revenue

The pharmaceutical industry systematically recruits former FDA officials for high-paying positions, creating powerful financial incentives for regulatory employees to maintain industry-friendly attitudes during their government service. This revolving door system ensures that regulatory decisions are made by people who expect to work for pharmaceutical companies in the future.

Former FDA officials often earn salaries that are multiples of their government pay when they join pharmaceutical companies, creating obvious financial motivations to avoid aggressive regulatory actions that might jeopardize future employment opportunities. The industry's recruitment of former regulators also provides companies with insider knowledge of regulatory processes and relationships that can be used to their advantage.

The Consulting Contract Web

Many regulatory officials maintain consulting relationships with pharmaceutical companies even while employed by government agencies, creating direct financial conflicts of interest in regulatory decision-making. These consulting arrangements often involve payments for speaking engagements, advisory committee participation, and research collaboration that can influence regulatory officials' perspectives on industry issues.

The consulting contract system allows pharmaceutical companies to develop financial relationships with regulators that create obligations and loyalties extending beyond official government responsibilities. These relationships can influence regulatory decisions in subtle ways that favor industry interests while maintaining the appearance of objective oversight.

The Clinical Trial Investment Scam

The pharmaceutical industry has developed sophisticated methods for conducting clinical trials that minimize safety oversight costs while maximizing regulatory approval chances, often at the expense of patient safety.

The Safety Endpoint Manipulation

Pharmaceutical companies design clinical trials with safety evaluation periods that are too short to detect long-term adverse effects, allowing them to gain regulatory approval based on limited safety data while avoiding the costs of extended safety monitoring. These abbreviated safety evaluations often miss serious adverse effects that only become apparent after years of patient use.

The manipulation of safety endpoints allows companies to present misleading safety profiles to regulators while technically complying with clinical trial requirements. Companies may focus on short-term safety metrics while ignoring longer-term risks that would be more costly to evaluate and might complicate regulatory approval.

The Patient Population Selection

Clinical trials typically exclude patients with complex medical conditions, multiple medications, or other factors that might increase adverse event risks, creating safety data that doesn't reflect real-world patient populations. This patient selection bias allows companies to present artificially favorable safety profiles while avoiding the costs and complications of testing in more representative patient groups.

The exclusion of complex patients from clinical trials means that post-market safety experience often differs significantly from pre-approval safety data, with real-world patients experiencing higher rates of adverse events than predicted from clinical trial results.

The Comparator Manipulation

Many clinical trials compare new medications to placebo rather than existing treatments, allowing companies to avoid demonstrating superior safety compared to available alternatives. This comparator manipulation reduces clinical trial costs while making it easier to achieve regulatory approval even when new medications offer no safety advantages over existing treatments.

Companies may also choose comparator medications that are known to have poor safety profiles, making their new products appear safer by comparison rather than demonstrating absolute safety advantages.

The Liability Shield System

The pharmaceutical industry has developed a sophisticated legal and financial infrastructure designed to minimize liability exposure from safety problems while maximizing profits from potentially dangerous products.

The Corporate Structure Protection

Pharmaceutical companies often structure their operations through complex networks of subsidiaries and shell companies that limit liability exposure when safety problems occur. These corporate structures allow companies to isolate manufacturing operations, research activities, and marketing functions in separate legal entities that can be abandoned if major liability issues arise.

When contamination or safety scandals emerge, companies can often blame subsidiaries or contractors while protecting parent company assets from legal exposure. This corporate structure manipulation allows companies to benefit from risky operations while limiting their financial exposure to the consequences.

The Insurance Cost Transfer

Pharmaceutical companies transfer liability risks to insurance companies and reinsurance markets, allowing them to continue risky operations while spreading potential costs across multiple financial entities. This risk transfer system often results in insurance companies rather than pharmaceutical companies paying settlements and judgments when safety problems cause patient harm.

The insurance system allows pharmaceutical companies to treat safety liability as a manageable business cost rather than a fundamental operational consideration, encouraging risk-taking behavior that might be modified if companies bore direct financial responsibility for safety failures.

The Settlement Secrecy Strategy

When safety problems do result in legal liability, pharmaceutical companies routinely negotiate settlement agreements that include secrecy provisions preventing public disclosure of safety information. These secrecy agreements allow companies to resolve individual legal cases while preventing the broader public from learning about safety risks that might affect other patients.

The settlement secrecy system means that important safety information discovered through litigation often never reaches other patients who might be at risk from the same products. This secrecy serves pharmaceutical company interests by preventing safety information from reaching potential plaintiffs or regulatory agencies.

The Political Investment Portfolio

The pharmaceutical industry maintains one of the largest and most sophisticated political lobbying and campaign contribution systems in American politics, designed to prevent regulatory reforms that might reduce industry profits.

The Legislative Purchase Program

Pharmaceutical companies and their trade associations spend hundreds of millions of dollars annually on lobbying activities designed to prevent legislation that would strengthen safety oversight or increase industry accountability. This lobbying investment often yields returns that far exceed the lobbying costs by preventing regulatory changes that might reduce industry profits.

The industry's lobbying efforts focus particularly on preventing laws that would increase inspection frequency, enhance recall requirements, or strengthen penalties for safety violations. These lobbying investments protect the industry's ability to continue current practices that prioritize profits over patient safety.

The Campaign Contribution Strategy

Pharmaceutical companies and their executives make substantial campaign contributions to legislators who serve on committees with oversight responsibilities for drug regulation and healthcare policy. These contributions create financial relationships that influence legislative decisions on pharmaceutical oversight and safety regulation.

The campaign contribution system ensures that legislators considering pharmaceutical safety legislation hear from well-funded industry representatives while patient advocacy groups typically lack comparable financial resources to influence legislative decisions.

The State-Level Influence Operations

The pharmaceutical industry has expanded its political influence operations to state and local levels, recognizing that these jurisdictions increasingly play important roles in pharmaceutical oversight and consumer protection. State-level lobbying often focuses on preventing local safety regulations that might be more stringent than federal requirements.

Industry influence at state levels can prevent local initiatives that might serve as models for national reform, maintaining the current federal system that provides minimal safety oversight while appearing to address public concerns about pharmaceutical safety.

The Academic Capture Investment

The pharmaceutical industry has systematically invested in academic institutions and research programs to ensure that academic research supports industry positions on safety and regulatory issues.

The Research Funding Influence

Pharmaceutical companies provide substantial funding to academic researchers and institutions, creating financial dependencies that can influence research priorities and outcomes. Academic researchers who receive industry funding may be reluctant to pursue research questions or publish results that could jeopardize future funding opportunities.

The industry's academic funding creates research environments where questions about pharmaceutical safety receive less attention than topics that support industry interests, skewing the overall body of scientific knowledge in favor of industry positions.

The Expert Witness Development

The pharmaceutical industry cultivates relationships with academic experts who can serve as witnesses in regulatory proceedings and legal cases, often providing these experts with consulting fees, research funding, and other financial benefits that create loyalties to industry positions.

These expert relationships ensure that industry positions receive academic credibility in regulatory and legal proceedings while making it difficult for patient advocates to find independent experts willing to challenge industry claims.

The Conference and Publication Sponsorship

Pharmaceutical companies sponsor academic conferences, scientific journals, and professional organizations that shape medical and scientific opinion on pharmaceutical issues. This sponsorship influence can affect which research gets presented, which safety concerns receive attention, and how regulatory issues are framed in professional discussions.

The sponsorship system creates academic environments where pharmaceutical industry positions receive favorable treatment while critical perspectives on industry practices may be marginalized or excluded from professional discourse.

The Patient Advocacy Corruption

The pharmaceutical industry has invested heavily in patient advocacy organizations, often co-opting groups that should represent patient interests to instead promote industry positions on safety and regulatory issues.

The Funding Dependency Creation

Many prominent patient advocacy organizations receive substantial funding from pharmaceutical companies, creating financial dependencies that influence these organizations' positions on regulatory and safety issues. Organizations that depend on industry funding may be reluctant to advocate for regulatory changes that could affect their financial supporters.

This funding dependency corrupts the patient advocacy landscape by ensuring that organizations claiming to represent patient interests often actually promote pharmaceutical industry positions rather than challenging industry practices that harm patients.

The Grassroots Manipulation

Pharmaceutical companies create and fund fake grassroots organizations that claim to represent patient interests while actually promoting industry positions on regulatory and safety issues. These astroturf organizations can influence regulatory proceedings and legislative debates by creating the appearance of patient support for industry positions.

The grassroots manipulation system allows pharmaceutical companies to present industry interests as patient interests, confusing public debates about pharmaceutical safety and regulation while maintaining the appearance of democratic participation in policy decisions.

The Access Argument Exploitation

The pharmaceutical industry has trained patient advocacy organizations to frame regulatory and safety issues in terms of "access" rather than safety, arguing that increased safety requirements will reduce patient access to medications. This framing shifts debates away from safety considerations toward access concerns that favor industry interests.

The access argument manipulation allows pharmaceutical companies to present safety regulations as threats to patient welfare rather than protections for patient safety, using patient advocacy organizations to oppose regulatory reforms that would actually protect patient interests.

The Breaking Point Economics

The current pharmaceutical safety crisis exists because the financial incentives that drive industry behavior consistently reward companies for exposing patients to unnecessary risks while punishing those who prioritize safety over profits.

The Profit-Safety Equation

Every major pharmaceutical safety scandal—from contaminated heparin to NDMA-tainted blood pressure medications—represents a situation where companies calculated that the financial benefits of risky practices outweighed the potential costs of safety problems. This profit-safety equation consistently favors risk-taking because the financial penalties for safety failures are typically much smaller than the profits generated by cost-cutting measures.

Until the financial costs of safety failures exceed the profits generated by risky practices, companies will continue to choose profits over patient safety because that choice is economically rational under current regulatory and legal systems.

The Systemic Change Requirement

Meaningful pharmaceutical safety reform will require fundamental changes in the financial incentives that drive industry behavior. These changes must make safety compliance more profitable than safety violations, and they must ensure that companies bear the full financial costs of safety failures rather than passing these costs on to patients and healthcare systems.

The current system socializes the costs of pharmaceutical safety failures while privatizing the profits from risky practices. Reform must reverse this equation by ensuring that companies pay the full costs of safety problems while reducing the financial benefits of safety violations.

The Reform Investment Return

The financial investment required to implement meaningful pharmaceutical safety reform would be substantial, but the economic returns from improved safety would far exceed these costs through reduced healthcare expenses, improved patient outcomes, and increased public confidence in medication safety.

The current system's hidden costs—including healthcare expenses from adverse events, lost productivity from medication-related health problems, and reduced medication compliance due to safety concerns—represent economic losses that far exceed the costs of implementing better safety systems.

Following the money trail through the pharmaceutical industry reveals a system designed to maximize profits while minimizing accountability for patient safety. Every aspect of pharmaceutical manufacturing, regulation, and distribution is structured to reward companies for cutting corners on safety while protecting them from the financial consequences of safety failures.

Until we acknowledge that the pharmaceutical safety crisis is fundamentally an economic problem created by financial incentives that reward dangerous practices, and until we implement reforms that make safety compliance more profitable than safety violations, patients will continue to serve as unwitting victims of an industry that treats their health as a cost to be minimized rather than a responsibility to be protected.

The next time you hear pharmaceutical companies claim they can't afford better safety measures, remember that these same companies spend billions on marketing, lobbying, and executive compensation while arguing that patient safety is too expensive to prioritize. The money is there—it's just being invested in protecting profits rather than protecting patients.

Chapter 12: Reading Between the Lines

After discovering the extensive contamination and deception that permeates the pharmaceutical industry, I realized that protecting myself and my family would require becoming a detective every time I encountered a medication. The comfortable assumption that someone else was ensuring medication safety had been shattered, replaced by the harsh reality that patients must advocate for themselves in a system designed to hide crucial information.

Learning to read between the lines of pharmaceutical marketing, labeling, and official communications became essential survival skills. The industry's sophisticated methods for concealing risks and manipulating information meant that protecting my health required understanding not just what companies say, but what they don't say, how they say it, and why they choose specific language to obscure rather than illuminate the truth.

This chapter will teach you the skills I developed through necessity—how to decode pharmaceutical communications, research medication safety, identify red flags that indicate potential problems, and ask the right questions to protect yourself from a system that profits from your ignorance. These aren't skills you should need, but in the current pharmaceutical landscape, they're absolutely essential for anyone who wants to make informed decisions about their health.

Decoding Pharmaceutical Language

The pharmaceutical industry has developed a sophisticated vocabulary designed to minimize apparent risks while maximizing perceived benefits. Learning to translate this corporate-speak is essential for understanding what companies are really telling you about their products.

The "Generally Recognized as Safe" Deception

When you see the term "Generally Recognized as Safe" (GRAS) on pharmaceutical labeling or marketing materials, understand that this doesn't mean the ingredient has been proven safe for pharmaceutical use. GRAS designation often means that the ingredient has been used in food or other applications without obvious immediate harm, but it may never have been tested for safety in the specific pharmaceutical application you're considering.

The GRAS designation allows companies to include ingredients that sound safe while avoiding the expense of actual safety testing. When you encounter GRAS claims, research the specific ingredient's history and ask whether safety testing has been conducted for your specific use case.

The "Clinical Studies Show" Manipulation

Pharmaceutical marketing frequently claims that "clinical studies show" numerous benefits or safety profiles, but these references are often misleading. Companies may reference studies that:

Were conducted by the company itself rather than independent researchers

Involved different patient populations than those who will use the medication

Measured different outcomes than what's being claimed in marketing

Used different dosages or formulations than the marketed product

Were conducted for such short periods that long-term effects couldn't be detected

When you encounter "clinical studies show" claims, demand specific references to peer-reviewed research and verify that the studies actually support the claims being made.

The "FDA Approved" Illusion

"FDA Approved" sounds definitive and reassuring, but this designation can be misleading depending on what specifically was approved and under what circumstances. FDA approval might refer to:

Only the active ingredient, not the complete formulation you're taking

Approval based on limited clinical trials that didn't include people like you

Approval for different conditions than what you're using the medication for

Approval that occurred decades ago under less stringent safety standards

Approval that has been modified or restricted since the original designation

Understanding the scope and limitations of FDA approval helps you make more informed decisions about whether a medication is appropriate for your specific situation.

The Risk Minimization Vocabulary

Pharmaceutical companies use specific language to minimize the apparent severity of risks and side effects:

"Rare" often means affecting 1 in 1,000 people, which isn't particularly rare if millions of people take the medication

"Mild" side effects can still significantly impact quality of life

"Temporary" effects might last weeks or months

"May cause" often means "definitely causes in some people"

"Associated with" is used to avoid claiming direct causation even when causation is clear

Learning to interpret this risk-minimization language helps you understand the real likelihood and potential severity of medication-related problems.

Investigating Medication Sources and Quality

Protecting yourself from contaminated or low-quality medications requires developing research skills that allow you to evaluate manufacturers, supply chains, and quality histories before choosing medications.

Researching Manufacturer Track Records

Before accepting any medication, research the manufacturer's history of quality problems, recalls, and regulatory violations. Key resources include:

FDA Warning Letters Database: Search for letters sent to your medication's manufacturer to identify recurring quality problems

FDA Inspection Reports: Review inspection findings for facilities that produce your medications

Recall Databases: Check whether the manufacturer has history of recalls for contamination or quality issues

News Archives: Search for news coverage of safety problems at manufacturing facilities

Pay particular attention to patterns of violations rather than isolated incidents. Manufacturers with multiple warning letters or recurring inspection problems may have systemic quality issues that increase your risk.

Tracing Supply Chain Origins

Understanding where your medications actually come from helps you assess quality and contamination risks:

Ask pharmacists about manufacturing origins: Many pharmacists can provide information about which facilities produced specific medication batches

Research parent company relationships: Generic medications may be produced by subsidiaries of larger companies with different quality standards

Identify contract manufacturing arrangements: Many medications are produced by contract manufacturers who may have different quality standards than the companies selling the products

Investigate raw material sourcing: Active ingredients and excipients may come from different suppliers with varying quality standards

Understanding the complete supply chain helps you make informed decisions about medication safety and quality.

Evaluating Generic Medication Quality

Generic medications require special scrutiny because quality can vary significantly between manufacturers:

Compare inactive ingredient lists: Different generic versions may contain different allergens and chemical additives

Research bioequivalence data: Some generic manufacturers provide more extensive bioequivalence testing than others

Check manufacturing facility histories: Generic facilities may have different inspection records and quality histories

Monitor your response to manufacturer changes: Track symptoms and effectiveness when your pharmacy switches between generic manufacturers

Maintaining detailed records of which generic manufacturers work best for you helps you request specific formulations and avoid problematic ones.

Reading Medication Labels Like a Detective

Pharmaceutical labeling contains crucial safety information, but companies often bury vital details in technical language or fine print that most patients never read carefully.

Decoding Inactive Ingredient Lists

The inactive ingredient list often contains more chemicals than the active ingredient section, yet most patients ignore this information entirely. Learning to decode these lists is essential for avoiding allergens and unnecessary chemical exposure:

Identify potential allergens: Look for lactose (dairy), soy lecithin (soy), wheat starch (gluten), and other common allergens hidden under chemical names

Recognize artificial additives: FD&C dyes, artificial flavors, and synthetic preservatives serve no medical purpose and may cause adverse reactions

Understand functional categories: Fillers, binders, lubricants, and coatings each serve manufacturing purposes but may affect how medications behave in your body

Research unfamiliar chemicals: Don't assume that unrecognizable chemical names represent safe substances

Keeping a personal list of ingredients that cause problems for you helps you quickly identify medications to avoid.

Understanding Expiration Date Manipulation

Medication expiration dates often reflect marketing considerations rather than actual safety or effectiveness limits:

Stability testing limitations: Expiration dates are based on limited testing periods and may not reflect actual medication lifespan

Storage condition assumptions: Expiration dates assume ideal storage conditions that may not reflect real-world use

Batch-to-batch variation: Different manufacturing batches may have different actual expiration characteristics

Regulatory minimum requirements: Some medications remain effective well beyond their expiration dates while others may degrade quickly

Understanding the limitations of expiration dating helps you make informed decisions about medication storage and replacement.

Identifying Warning Sign Language

Medication labeling often contains subtle warning signs that indicate potential problems:

Extensive contraindication lists: Medications with long lists of conditions that preclude use may have broad safety concerns

Vague side effect descriptions: Medications that list "other effects" or "additional reactions" may have poorly understood safety profiles

Complex dosing instructions: Medications requiring elaborate dosing schedules may have narrow therapeutic windows or significant interaction risks

Multiple strength formulations: Medications available in many different strengths may be difficult to dose appropriately or may have significant toxicity risks

Learning to recognize these warning signs helps you identify medications that may require extra caution or medical supervision.

Researching Safety Information Beyond Official Sources

Pharmaceutical companies and regulatory agencies control most official medication information, making independent research essential for understanding real-world safety profiles and patient experiences.

Accessing Independent Research Databases

Several databases provide access to independent research that may not appear in official pharmaceutical communications:

PubMed: Search for peer-reviewed research on medication safety, contamination, and adverse effects

Cochrane Reviews: Access systematic reviews that analyze multiple studies on medication effectiveness and safety

Clinical Trial Registries: Review original clinical trial data rather than relying on company summaries

International Safety Databases: Research safety information from regulatory agencies in other countries that may have different standards

Independent research often reveals safety concerns that don't appear in official pharmaceutical marketing or labeling.

Learning from Patient Experience Networks

Patient-reported experiences can provide valuable safety information that doesn't appear in clinical trials or official reporting systems:

Patient advocacy organization databases: Many organizations maintain databases of patient-reported adverse effects and experiences

Online patient communities: Forums and support groups often discuss real-world medication experiences and problems

Social media monitoring: Patients often share medication experiences on social platforms before problems are officially recognized

Healthcare provider networks: Some healthcare providers maintain informal networks for sharing patient safety observations

Patient experience data helps identify safety patterns that may not be captured in formal reporting systems.

Monitoring International Safety Information

Safety information from other countries can provide early warnings about problems that haven't yet been addressed by American regulators:

European Medicines Agency alerts: European safety communications often precede American actions

Health Canada advisories: Canadian safety warnings may identify problems not yet addressed in the US

WHO safety communications: World Health Organization alerts may identify global safety patterns

Academic international research: Research from other countries may identify safety concerns not studied in American research

International safety monitoring helps identify potential problems before they're officially recognized in American regulatory systems.

Asking the Right Questions

Protecting yourself from pharmaceutical dangers requires asking specific questions that healthcare providers and pharmacists may not volunteer to address.

Questions for Healthcare Providers

When medications are prescribed, ask specific questions that force consideration of safety factors beyond basic effectiveness:

"What specific manufacturer and facility will produce this medication?"

"What alternatives are available if I experience problems with inactive ingredients?"

"How will we monitor for long-term effects that weren't studied in clinical trials?"

"What's the contamination and recall history for this medication?"

"Are there safer alternatives that might be equally effective?"

These questions force healthcare providers to consider safety factors they might otherwise ignore and help you make more informed treatment decisions.

Questions for Pharmacists

Pharmacists often have access to safety information that they don't routinely share with patients:

"Which generic manufacturer will you use, and can I request a specific one?"

"What's the recall history for this medication and manufacturer?"

"What inactive ingredients should I be concerned about?"

"How should I monitor for contamination or quality problems?"

"What symptoms might indicate problems with medication quality?"

Pharmacists can often provide detailed safety information if you ask specific questions rather than acccpting routine counseling.

Questions for Insurance Companies

Insurance coverage decisions often prioritize cost over safety, but you can advocate for safer alternatives by asking the right questions:

"What's the safety difference between the covered medication and alternatives?"

"What documentation do you need to cover a safer alternative?"

"How do I appeal coverage decisions based on safety concerns?"

"What's your policy for covering brand-name medications when generics cause problems?"

Understanding insurance policies and appeal processes helps you access safer medications when standard coverage creates safety risks.

Building Your Personal Safety Database

Protecting yourself from pharmaceutical dangers requires maintaining detailed records that help you identify patterns and make informed decisions about future medication use.

Tracking Your Medication History

Maintain detailed records of your medication experiences including:

Specific manufacturers and lot numbers: This information helps you identify patterns when problems occur

Symptom timelines: Track when symptoms start and stop in relation to medication changes

Effectiveness variations: Note differences in medication effectiveness that might indicate quality problems

Side effect patterns: Document adverse effects that might be related to inactive ingredients rather than active drugs

Pharmacy and supply chain changes: Track when your pharmacy switches suppliers or manufacturers

Detailed medication records help you identify patterns that healthcare providers might miss and make informed decisions about future medication choices.

Monitoring Recall and Safety Alerts

Develop systems for staying informed about recalls and safety alerts that might affect your medications:

Set up automated alerts: Use FDA and manufacturer websites to receive automatic notifications about recalls

Regular database searches: Periodically search recall databases for medications you take regularly

Healthcare provider communication: Establish systems with your healthcare providers for communicating about recall information

Pharmacy notification systems: Ensure your pharmacy has current contact information and will notify you about recalls

Staying informed about recalls and safety alerts helps you respond quickly when problems are identified.

Creating Your Personal Risk Profile

Develop a comprehensive understanding of your personal risk factors that might make you more vulnerable to medication problems:

Known allergies and sensitivities: Maintain detailed lists of substances that cause problems for you

Medication interaction history: Track combinations that have caused problems in the past

Underlying health conditions: Understand how your health conditions might affect medication metabolism and safety

Genetic factors: Consider genetic testing that might identify medication metabolism differences

Environmental exposures: Track other chemical exposures that might interact with medications

Understanding your personal risk profile helps you make informed decisions about medication safety and communicate effectively with healthcare providers.

Advocating for Transparency and Safety

Individual patients have more power than they realize to demand better safety information and practices from healthcare providers, pharmacists, and pharmaceutical companies.

Demanding Better Information

Don't accept vague or inadequate safety information from healthcare providers or pharmaceutical companies:

Request specific safety data: Ask for detailed information about contamination risks, quality problems, and long-term effects

Demand alternative options: Insist on information about safer alternatives when safety concerns exist

Require clear explanations: Don't accept technical jargon or dismissive responses to legitimate safety questions

Document safety concerns: Maintain written records of safety discussions and decisions

Demanding better information forces healthcare providers and companies to take safety concerns seriously and provides documentation for future advocacy.

Building Healthcare Provider Accountability

Healthcare providers who prescribe medications have professional obligations to consider patient safety that you can help enforce:

Request documentation of safety discussions: Ask for written summaries of safety considerations in treatment decisions

Demand consideration of alternatives: Insist that providers explain why they're recommending specific medications over safer alternatives

Report inadequate safety counseling: File complaints with medical boards when providers fail to address legitimate safety concerns

Seek second opinions: Consult additional providers when you're not satisfied with safety explanations

Building accountability helps ensure that healthcare providers take safety considerations seriously in treatment decisions.

Supporting Systemic Reform

Individual advocacy can contribute to broader reform efforts that improve safety for all patients:

Contact legislators: Advocate for stronger safety regulations and oversight requirements

Support patient advocacy organizations: Join organizations working for pharmaceutical safety reform

Share your experiences: Contribute to databases and research efforts that document patient experiences with medication safety

Educate others: Help other patients develop the skills needed to protect themselves from pharmaceutical dangers

Individual advocacy efforts can contribute to systemic changes that improve safety for all patients.

The Technology Tools for Safety

Modern technology provides powerful tools for researching medication safety and monitoring for problems that weren't available to previous generations of patients.

Mobile Apps and Databases

Several smartphone apps and online databases can help you research medication safety and track your experiences:

Drug interaction checkers: Apps that identify potential interactions between medications, supplements, and foods

Recall monitoring systems: Services that alert you when medications you take are recalled

Side effect databases: Platforms where patients report and research medication experiences

Manufacturer tracking tools: Apps that help you identify which companies produced your medications

Technology tools can automate much of the research and monitoring needed to protect yourself from medication dangers.

Electronic Health Record Integration

Many healthcare systems now provide patient access to electronic health records that can help you monitor your medication safety:

Medication lists with lot numbers: Some systems track specific medication batches you've received

Allergy and sensitivity tracking: Electronic systems can help you maintain comprehensive allergy profiles

Drug interaction monitoring: Electronic prescribing systems may identify potential interactions

Communication tools: Patient portals allow you to communicate safety concerns with healthcare providers

Electronic health records can provide valuable tools for monitoring and communicating about medication safety.

Social Media and Online Communities

Online platforms provide access to real-time information about medication experiences and safety concerns:

Patient community forums: Platforms where patients share experiences with specific medications and manufacturers

Healthcare provider networks: Social platforms where healthcare providers discuss medication safety observations

Real-time safety monitoring: social media can provide early warnings about safety problems before official alerts

Advocacy network organization: Online platforms help organize patient advocacy for safety improvements

Online communities can provide valuable safety information and support for patients navigating medication safety challenges.

Learning to read between the lines of pharmaceutical communications is essential for protecting yourself in a system designed to prioritize profits over patient safety. The skills outlined in this chapter—decoding corporate language, researching manufacturer quality, reading labels carefully, asking the right questions, and building personal safety databases—represent the minimum competencies needed to navigate safely through the modern pharmaceutical landscape.

These aren't skills you should need to develop, but given the current state of pharmaceutical safety oversight, they're absolutely essential for anyone who wants to make informed decisions about their health. The industry's sophisticated methods for concealing risks and manipulating information mean that your safety depends on your ability to see through deception and demand transparency.

The time you invest in developing these skills will pay dividends in better health outcomes and increased confidence in your medication decisions. More importantly, your individual advocacy for transparency and safety contributes to broader reform efforts that can improve protection for all patients.

Remember that you have more power than you realize to demand better information and safer practices from the healthcare system. Use that power to protect yourself and your family and help build a system that prioritizes patient safety over pharmaceutical profits.

Chapter 13: Minimizing Your Risk

After everything I've learned about pharmaceutical contamination, hidden chemicals, and regulatory failures, people often ask me whether I've stopped taking medications entirely. The answer is no—but I've fundamentally changed how I approach medication decisions. Instead of blindly trusting the system, I now treat every medication choice as a calculated risk-benefit analysis where I'm the final decision-maker, not a passive recipient of whatever healthcare providers and insurance companies decide is convenient.

Minimizing your risk from pharmaceutical dangers doesn't mean avoiding all medications or embracing medical conspiracy theories. It means becoming an informed consumer who understands the real risks and benefits of medication choices, who demands transparency from healthcare providers and pharmaceutical companies, and who takes active responsibility for protecting their own health within a flawed system.

The strategies I've developed through necessity—from my 18 surgeries and subsequent discoveries about hidden soy and dairy—represent practical approaches that any patient can implement to reduce their exposure to pharmaceutical dangers while still accessing the medical care they need. These aren't extreme measures; they're common-sense precautions that should be standard practice in a system that truly prioritized patient safety.

Developing Your Personal Risk Assessment Framework

The first step in minimizing pharmaceutical risks is developing a systematic approach to evaluating medication choices that considers factors beyond basic effectiveness and cost.

Understanding Your Individual Vulnerability Profile

Not all patients face equal risks from pharmaceutical dangers. Your personal vulnerability depends on multiple factors that should influence every medication decision:

Age-Related Factors: Children and elderly patients process medications differently than healthy adults and may be more vulnerable to contamination and chemical additives. Pediatric patients face higher dose-per-kilogram exposures to inactive ingredients, while elderly patients may have reduced ability to eliminate toxic substances.

Health Status Considerations: Patients with compromised immune systems, liver problems, kidney disease, or chronic illnesses may be more susceptible to pharmaceutical contamination and adverse effects from chemical additives. Your underlying health conditions should influence both medication choices and monitoring strategies.

Genetic Factors: Individual genetic variations affect how people metabolize medications and respond to chemical exposures. Consider genetic testing for medication metabolism if you've experienced unusual responses to standard medications or have family history of medication sensitivity.

Multiple Medication Interactions: Patients taking several medications simultaneously face compound risks from chemical additives, contamination, and drug interactions that aren't routinely evaluated. The more medications you take, the more important it becomes to minimize unnecessary chemical exposures.

Environmental and Lifestyle Factors: Your occupation, location, diet, and lifestyle choices affect your overall chemical exposure burden and may influence how you respond to pharmaceutical additives and contaminants.

Creating Your Personal Risk-Benefit Calculator

For every medication decision, develop a systematic evaluation process that weighs real risks against actual benefits:

Severity Assessment: How serious is the condition being treated? Life-threatening conditions may justify accepting higher pharmaceutical risks than minor symptoms that could be managed through other approaches.

Efficacy Evidence: What's the actual evidence that the medication will help your specific situation? Demand specific information about effectiveness in patients like you rather than accepting general population data.

Alternative Options: What other treatment approaches are available? Consider non-pharmaceutical interventions, lifestyle modifications, or safer medication alternatives before accepting high-risk options.

Time Sensitivity: How urgent is treatment? Acute conditions may require accepting immediate risks, while chronic conditions allow time for careful evaluation of safer approaches.

Reversibility: Can medication effects be easily reversed if problems occur? Some medications create permanent changes that can't be undone if adverse effects develop.

Implementing Medication Safety Protocols

Protecting yourself from pharmaceutical dangers requires establishing systematic safety protocols that you follow consistently regardless of pressure from healthcare providers or insurance companies.

The Brand Name vs. Generic Decision Matrix

Generic medications present unique risks that require careful evaluation:

When to Choose Brand Names:

Medications with narrow therapeutic indexes where small variations in bioequivalence could cause dangerous effects

Medications you'll take long-term where consistency is more important than cost savings

Situations where you've had problems with generic formulations in the past

Critical medications where treatment failure could have grave consequences

When Generics May Be Acceptable:

Short-term use where minor variations in effectiveness won't have long-term consequences

Medications with wide therapeutic windows where bioequivalence variations are less dangerous

Situations where you can closely monitor effectiveness and switch if problems occur

Cases where the cost difference makes brand names financially impossible

The Manufacturer Selection Strategy

When using generic medications, develop strategies for selecting and maintaining consistency with higher-quality manufacturers:

Research Manufacturer Quality Histories: Before accepting any generic medication, research the manufacturer's FDA inspection records, warning letter history, and recall frequency. Choose manufacturers with better safety records when options are available.

Request Specific Manufacturers: Many pharmacies can order medications from specific manufacturers if you request this service. Establish relationships with pharmacists who will work with you to maintain manufacturer consistency.

Monitor Quality Indicators: Track your response to different manufacturers and maintain detailed records of which formulations work best for you. Use this information to make informed requests for specific manufacturers.

Avoid Problem Manufacturers: Maintain a personal blacklist of manufacturers that have caused problems for you or have poor safety records. Share this information with healthcare providers and pharmacists to prevent accidental exposure.

Optimizing Healthcare Provider Relationships

Protecting yourself from pharmaceutical dangers requires building relationships with healthcare providers who prioritize safety over convenience and who will work with you to minimize unnecessary risks.

Selecting Safety-Conscious Providers

Not all healthcare providers are equally committed to pharmaceutical safety. Look for providers who demonstrate genuine concern for medication safety:

Safety-Focused Interview Questions: When selecting healthcare providers, ask specific questions about their approach to medication safety:

"How do you evaluate the safety of generic vs. brand name medications?"

"What's your process for monitoring pharmaceutical recalls and safety alerts?"

"How do you handle patients who have concerns about inactive ingredients?"

"What's your approach to minimizing polypharmacy risks?"

Red Flag Warning Signs: Avoid healthcare providers who dismiss safety concerns, pressure you to accept specific medications without discussion, refuse to consider alternatives when safety issues exist, or seem more concerned with insurance formulary compliance than patient safety.

Collaborative Decision-Making Indicators: Look for providers who involve you in medication decisions, explain their reasoning for specific choices, respect your concerns about safety issues, and are willing to modify treatment approaches when problems occur.

Building Effective Communication Protocols

Establish clear communication systems with healthcare providers that ensure safety considerations are always part of medication decisions:

Pre-Visit Preparation: Before appointments, prepare specific questions about medication safety, research alternatives to medications being considered, gather information about your previous medication experiences, and bring lists of manufacturers or formulations that have worked well for you.

Documentation Requirements: Request written summaries of medication decisions including rationale for specific choices, safety considerations that were evaluated, alternative options that were considered, and monitoring plans for detecting problems.

Follow-Up Systems: Establish clear protocols for communicating about medication problems, reporting adverse effects or concerns, requesting medication changes when issues occur, and accessing urgent consultation when safety problems arise.

Second Opinion Strategies: Know when and how to seek second opinions, especially for medications with significant safety risks, long-term treatment decisions, situations where you're not satisfied with safety explanations, or cases involving expensive or potentially dangerous medications.

Minimizing Contamination and Quality Risks

Given the widespread contamination problems in pharmaceutical manufacturing, develop specific strategies for reducing your exposure to contaminated or low-quality medications.

Supply Chain Risk Management

Understanding and managing pharmaceutical supply chain risks requires active investigation and monitoring:

Manufacturer Facility Research: For medications you take regularly, research the specific facilities where they're manufactured. Check FDA inspection records, warning letter histories, and recall patterns for these facilities.

Supply Chain Transparency: Ask pharmacists and healthcare providers about medication supply chains. Request information about raw material sources, manufacturing locations, and distribution pathways.

Geographic Risk Assessment: Understand that medications manufactured in certain countries may carry higher contamination risks due to environmental pollution, less stringent regulatory oversight, or lower manufacturing standards.

Timing and Storage Optimization: Minimize contamination risks through proper medication storage, rotation of medication supplies to avoid expired products, awareness of storage conditions that might increase contamination risks, and timing of medication purchases to avoid potentially problematic batches.

Quality Monitoring Strategies

Develop systematic approaches for monitoring medication quality and detecting potential problems:

Physical Inspection Protocols: Regularly inspect medications for changes in appearance, unusual odors or tastes, particles or discoloration, damaged packaging or seals, and any other indicators of potential quality problems.

Effectiveness Monitoring: Track medication effectiveness over time to identify potential quality problems. Sudden changes in effectiveness might indicate contamination or quality degradation rather than disease progression.

Side Effect Pattern Recognition: Monitor for new or unusual side effects that might indicate contamination rather than normal medication effects. Keep detailed records of symptom timing and patterns.

Batch Number Tracking: Maintain records of specific batch numbers for medications you take, especially for long-term medications. This information is crucial if recalls occur or if you need to identify problematic batches.

Creating Medication-Free Zones and Alternatives

Minimizing pharmaceutical risks often involves reducing your overall medication burden through lifestyle modifications and alternative approaches that address underlying health issues.

Lifestyle Interventions That Reduce Medication Dependence

Many health conditions that require pharmaceutical treatment can be improved through lifestyle modifications that reduce medication needs:

Cardiovascular Health: Diet modifications, exercise programs, stress management, and weight control can often reduce or eliminate the need for blood pressure and cholesterol medications while providing better long-term health outcomes.

Diabetes Management: Dietary changes, weight management, and exercise can significantly improve blood sugar control and may reduce medication requirements for many people with type 2 diabetes.

Mental Health Support: Therapy, stress management, social support, and lifestyle modifications can often reduce dependence on psychiatric medications while providing more sustainable mental health improvements.

Pain Management: Physical therapy, exercise, stress reduction, and other non-pharmaceutical approaches can often provide better long-term pain relief than medication-dependent strategies.

Sleep Optimization: Sleep hygiene, stress management, and addressing underlying sleep disorders can often eliminate the need for sleep medications while providing better-quality rest.

Supplement and Nutritional Approaches

While supplements aren't always safer than pharmaceuticals, they may provide lower-risk alternatives for some health conditions:

Quality Supplement Selection: Choose supplements from manufacturers with good quality control records, third-party testing verification, minimal unnecessary additives, and transparent sourcing information.

Evidence-Based Choices: Focus on supplements with solid research support rather than marketing claims. Prioritize interventions with compelling evidence for safety and effectiveness.

Professional Guidance: Work with healthcare providers who understand both pharmaceutical and nutritional approaches to health. Avoid providers who dismiss either pharmaceutical or nutritional interventions entirely.

Monitoring and Safety: Apply the same safety monitoring principles to supplements that you use for pharmaceuticals. Supplements can cause adverse effects and interact with other medications.

Emergency Preparedness and Crisis Management

Despite your best efforts to minimize pharmaceutical risks, you may occasionally face situations where you need medications despite safety concerns, or where you experience problems with medications you're already taking.

Developing Crisis Protocols

Prepare for situations where you may need to make rapid medication decisions under less-than-ideal circumstances:

Emergency Medication Lists: Maintain updated lists of medications that are acceptable for emergency use, including specific manufacturers and formulations when possible. Share these lists with emergency contacts and healthcare providers.

Alternative Emergency Treatments: Research and discuss with healthcare providers what alternative treatments might be available if standard emergency medications are problematic for you.

Communication Strategies: Develop systems for communicating medication sensitivities and safety concerns to emergency healthcare providers who may not know your medical history.

Documentation Accessibility: Ensure that information about your medication sensitivities, allergies, and safety concerns is easily accessible to healthcare providers in emergency situations.

Managing Medication Problems

When problems occur with medications you're already taking, have clear protocols for response:

Problem Recognition: Develop skills for recognizing when new symptoms might be related to medication issues rather than disease progression or other factors.

Healthcare Provider Communication: Establish clear protocols for quickly communicating medication problems to healthcare providers and getting rapid responses to safety concerns.

Medication Discontinuation: Understand which medications can be safely stopped immediately when problems occur and which require gradual discontinuation under medical supervision.

Alternative Treatment Access: Know how to quickly access alternative treatments when medications need to be discontinued due to safety problems.

Building Support Networks for Medication Safety

Protecting yourself from pharmaceutical dangers is easier when your part of a community of informed patients who share information and support each other's efforts to maintain medication safety.

Patient Advocacy and Information Networks

Connect with other patients who prioritize medication safety and share information about effective strategies:

Online Communities: Participate in online forums and social media groups focused on medication safety and patient advocacy. Share your experiences and learn from others who have faced similar challenges.

Local Support Groups: Look for local patient advocacy groups or support organizations that focus on medication safety and healthcare transparency.

Professional Networks: Build relationships with healthcare providers, pharmacists, and other professionals who prioritize patient safety and medication transparency.

Information Sharing: Contribute to databases and research efforts that track patient experiences with medication safety and help other patients make informed decisions.

Family and Personal Support Systems

Educate family members and close friends about medication safety so they can support your efforts and advocate for you when necessary:

Education and Awareness: Help family members understand pharmaceutical safety issues and your specific concerns and strategies.

Emergency Advocacy: Train family members to advocate for your medication safety concerns in emergency situations when you might not be able to communicate effectively.

Information Management: Share medication safety information and documentation with trusted family members who can help manage your healthcare in crisis situations.

Decision Support: Include trusted family members or friends in important medication decisions, especially when dealing with complex safety considerations.

Long-Term Strategies for Pharmaceutical Independence

The ultimate goal of medication risk minimization is reducing your dependence on a pharmaceutical system that prioritizes profits over patient safety while maintaining access to genuinely beneficial medical interventions.

Preventive Health Strategies

Invest in preventive health approaches that reduce your likelihood of needing pharmaceutical interventions:

Regular Health Monitoring: Maintain regular health screenings and monitoring that can detect problems early when they're more amenable to non-pharmaceutical interventions.

Lifestyle Optimization: Continuously work on diet, exercise, stress management, and other lifestyle factors that reduce disease risk and medication dependence.

Environmental Health: Minimize exposure to environmental toxins and chemicals that might contribute to health problems requiring pharmaceutical treatment.

Social and Mental Health: Maintain strong social connections and mental health practices that reduce risk of conditions requiring psychiatric medications.

Knowledge and Skill Development

Continuously develop your knowledge and skills related to health and medication safety:

Ongoing Education: Stay informed about developments in medication safety, pharmaceutical industry practices, and patient advocacy efforts.

Research Skills: Develop and maintain skills for researching medication safety and making informed healthcare decisions.

Communication Skills: Improve your ability to communicate effectively with healthcare providers and advocate for your safety concerns.

Network Building: Continuously expand your network of safety-conscious healthcare providers, informed patients, and advocacy resources.

Minimizing your risk from pharmaceutical dangers requires treating medication decisions as serious safety choices rather than routine healthcare procedures. The strategies outlined in this chapter represent practical approaches that any patient can implement to protect themselves while still accessing necessary medical care.

These approaches require more time, effort, and vigilance than simply accepting whatever healthcare providers and insurance companies recommend, but the investment is worthwhile for anyone who wants to maintain control over their health and safety. The pharmaceutical industry's systematic prioritization of profits over patient safety means that your safety ultimately depends on your own knowledge, vigilance, and advocacy.

Remember that you have the right to make informed decisions about your healthcare, including the right to refuse medications that you believe pose unnecessary risks. Use that right wisely but use it. Your health and safety are too important to entrust entirely to a system that has repeatedly demonstrated that it cannot be trusted to prioritize patient welfare over corporate profits.

The International Options Strategy

One of the most effective ways to minimize pharmaceutical risks is understanding how to access safer medication options from countries with more stringent regulatory standards and quality control requirements.

Researching International Safety Standards

Different countries maintain varying levels of pharmaceutical oversight that can affect medication safety and quality:

European Union Standards: European medications often undergo more rigorous safety testing for inactive ingredients and maintain stricter contamination limits than American equivalents. The European Medicines Agency requires more comprehensive safety documentation and faster recall procedures.

Canadian Regulatory Advantages: Canadian pharmaceutical regulations include enhanced labeling requirements for allergens, more frequent facility inspections, and stricter quality control standards for generic medications.

Japanese Quality Systems: Japan maintains some of the world's most stringent pharmaceutical manufacturing standards, with mandatory contamination testing protocols that exceed American requirements.

Swiss Manufacturing Excellence: Swiss pharmaceutical facilities often maintain quality standards that exceed regulatory minimums, focusing on contamination prevention and quality consistency.

Legal Medication Importation

Understanding legal options for accessing international medications can provide safer alternatives when domestic options carry unacceptable risks:

Personal Importation Rules: FDA regulations allow personal importation of medications for individual use under specific circumstances, including situations where domestic alternatives pose safety risks or are unavailable.

Prescription Tourism: Some patients choose to fill prescriptions in countries with higher manufacturing standards, particularly for long-term medications where quality consistency is crucial.

International Pharmacy Networks: Several legitimate international pharmacy networks provide access to medications manufactured under different regulatory standards, though patients must carefully verify legitimacy and quality.

Healthcare Provider Coordination: Some healthcare providers can help coordinate access to international medications when safety concerns justify the additional complexity and cost.

Advanced Contamination Detection Strategies

Developing sophisticated methods for detecting contamination and quality problems can help you identify dangerous medications before they cause harm.

Home Testing Capabilities

Several testing approaches can help detect medication quality problems:

Visual Inspection Protocols: Develop systematic approaches for inspecting medications using magnification tools, consistent lighting conditions, comparison with reference samples, and photographic documentation of changes over time.

Dissolution Testing: Simple dissolution tests can help identify medications that may not perform as expected, though these tests require some technical knowledge and equipment.

Third-Party Testing Services: Some laboratories offer testing services for patients concerned about medication quality, though these services can be expensive and may not be covered by insurance.

Home Test Kits: Limited home testing options are available for detecting certain types of contamination, though these tests are not comprehensive and should be used as supplements to other safety strategies.

Professional Testing Networks

Building relationships with testing professionals can provide access to more sophisticated contamination detection:

Independent Laboratory Services: Some independent laboratories specialize in pharmaceutical testing and can provide detailed analysis of medication quality and contamination.

Academic Research Partnerships: University laboratories sometimes accept samples for research purposes, providing detailed analysis while contributing to pharmaceutical safety research.

Professional Consultation: Pharmaceutical chemists and quality control professionals sometimes provide consultation services for patients with specific contamination concerns.

Legal Testing Requirements: Understanding when medication testing might be legally required or supported can help access professional testing services through legal or insurance channels.

The Financial Strategies for Safer Medications

Accessing safer medications often requires navigating complex financial considerations and insurance limitations.

Insurance Advocacy Techniques

Developing sophisticated insurance advocacy skills can help access safer medications when standard coverage creates risks:

Medical Necessity Documentation: Work with healthcare providers to document medical necessity for specific manufacturers or formulations when safety considerations support these choices.

Appeal Process Optimization: Understand your insurance company's appeal processes and how to present safety-based arguments for coverage of non-formulary medications.

Prior Authorization Strategies: Develop efficient approaches for obtaining prior authorizations for safer alternatives when standard formulary options pose risks.

External Review Options: Know when and how to request external reviews of insurance coverage decisions, particularly when safety considerations support coverage of more expensive alternatives.

Cost-Benefit Financial Planning

Understanding the true costs of pharmaceutical choices helps make informed decisions about safety investments:

Total Cost Assessment: Calculate the complete fiscal impact of medication choices, including direct costs, potential adverse event expenses, monitoring requirements, and long-term health implications.

Safety Investment Prioritization: Develop strategies for prioritizing safety investments when financial resources are limited, focusing on medications with highest risk profiles or longest-term use requirements.

Alternative Funding Sources: Research patient assistance programs, manufacturer coupons, charitable foundations, and other funding sources that might help access safer medications.

Insurance Optimization: Understand how different insurance plans handle medication safety issues and factor this into insurance selection decisions.

Building Personal Medicine Expertise

Developing deep knowledge about your specific medications and health conditions provides the foundation for effective risk minimization.

Pharmacology Self-Education

Understanding how your medications actually work helps you make better safety decisions:

Mechanism of Action Knowledge: Learn how your medications work in your body and what factors might affect their safety and effectiveness.

Metabolism Pathway Understanding: Understand how your body processes your medications and what factors might affect these processes.

Interaction Recognition: Develop knowledge about how your medications might interact with foods, supplements, other medications, and environmental factors.

Individual Response Patterns: Learn to recognize your personal response patterns to different medications and manufacturers.

Quality Control Understanding

Developing knowledge about pharmaceutical manufacturing and quality control helps you evaluate medication safety:

Manufacturing Process Awareness: Understand how your medications are manufactured and what factors might affect quality and safety.

Quality Indicator Recognition: Learn to recognize signs of quality problems and manufacturing defects that might indicate safety concerns.

Supply Chain Knowledge: Understand the supply chain for your medications and how changes might affect quality and safety.

Regulatory Process Understanding: Develop knowledge about how pharmaceutical regulation works and where gaps might affect your medication safety.

The goal isn't to become paranoid about all medications, but to become an informed, empowered patient who makes thoughtful decisions based on real risks and benefits rather than marketing claims and system convenience. That transformation from passive patient to active advocate is the most major step you can take to protect yourself and your family from pharmaceutical dangers.

Chapter 14: The Path Forward

When I began this journey following my 18 surgeries and the discovery of hidden soy and dairy in my medications, I thought I was investigating a personal health problem. What I uncovered was a systematic betrayal of public trust that affects every American who takes medications—which is virtually all of us at some point in our lives.

The pharmaceutical industry has built a system that socializes the health risks of their cost-cutting measures while privatizing the profits from those same dangerous practices. They've captured regulatory agencies, corrupted academic research, co-opted patient advocacy organizations, and manipulated political processes to ensure that their right to profit takes precedence over our right to safe medications.

But this system isn't inevitable, and it isn't permanent. Other countries have proven that pharmaceutical manufacturing can prioritize patient safety without destroying industry profitability. International examples demonstrate that rigorous oversight, transparent manufacturing, and genuine accountability are not only possible but economically sustainable. The question isn't whether we can build a better system—it's whether we have the political will to demand one.

The path forward requires acknowledging that pharmaceutical safety is fundamentally a political problem that demands political solutions. Individual patients can protect themselves through the strategies outlined in previous chapters, but systemic change requires collective action that forces fundamental reforms in how medications are manufactured, regulated, and distributed in America.

The International Models That Work

Before designing solutions for America's pharmaceutical safety crisis, we should examine countries that have successfully balanced industry profitability with genuine patient protection.

The European Union's Precautionary Approach

The European Medicines Agency operates under a precautionary principle that requires pharmaceutical companies to prove safety rather than requiring regulators to prove harm. This fundamental shift in burden of proof has created a pharmaceutical environment where:

Enhanced Safety Testing: European regulations require specific safety testing for inactive ingredients, not just active compounds. Companies must demonstrate that every component of their medications is safe for pharmaceutical use rather than relying on general safety assumptions.

Stricter Contamination Limits: European contamination limits for pharmaceutical manufacturing are often 10-100 times more stringent than American standards, reflecting a genuine commitment to preventing patient exposure to harmful substances.

Mandatory Transparency: European pharmaceutical companies must disclose detailed manufacturing information, including facility locations, supply chain details, and quality control procedures. This transparency enables meaningful regulatory oversight and public accountability.

Rapid Response Systems: European recall and safety alert systems prioritize patient notification over industry convenience, with mandatory direct patient notification requirements and clear communication standards that ensure patients understand safety risks.

Real Enforcement Authority: European regulators have the authority to immediately halt operations at facilities with safety problems and can impose financial penalties that actually deter dangerous practices rather than treating them as acceptable business costs.

Canada's Balanced Oversight Model

Canada has developed pharmaceutical oversight systems that maintain industry competitiveness while providing stronger patient protection than American systems:

Enhanced Inspection Frequency: Canadian facilities receive more frequent inspections than American facilities, with mandatory unannounced inspections that observe actual operating conditions rather than carefully prepared presentations.

Supply Chain Transparency: Canadian regulations require pharmaceutical companies to maintain detailed supply chain documentation that enables rapid identification of contamination sources and quality problems.

Generic Quality Standards: Canada maintains higher quality standards for generic medications, with mandatory bioequivalence testing that goes beyond American requirements and stricter manufacturing oversight.

Patient-Centered Communication: Canadian recall and safety communication systems prioritize patient understanding over legal liability protection, with plain language requirements and mandatory patient notification procedures.

Switzerland's Manufacturing Excellence Standards

Switzerland has developed pharmaceutical manufacturing standards that demonstrate how rigorous oversight can coexist with industry innovation and profitability:

Voluntary Quality Excellence: Swiss pharmaceutical companies often exceed regulatory requirements because market reputation for quality provides competitive advantages that justify additional safety investments.

Environmental Integration: Swiss manufacturing standards integrate environmental protection with patient safety, recognizing that contaminated manufacturing environments produce contaminated medications.

Long-term Perspective: Swiss pharmaceutical regulation takes a long-term view of industry sustainability that recognizes genuine safety as essential for maintaining public trust and market stability.

Innovation Through Safety: Swiss companies have demonstrated that innovation in safety technology and quality control can provide competitive advantages while improving patient outcomes.

The Regulatory Reforms We Need

Transforming American pharmaceutical oversight requires comprehensive regulatory reforms that prioritize patient safety over industry convenience and political expediency.

Fundamental Structural Changes

American pharmaceutical regulation needs structural reforms that eliminate conflicts of interest and create genuine accountability:

Independent Funding: The FDA's pharmaceutical oversight operations should be funded through general taxation rather than user fees paid by pharmaceutical companies. This funding independence would eliminate the obvious conflict of interest where regulators depend financially on the industries they're supposed to police.

Revolving Door Restrictions: Comprehensive restrictions on movement between regulatory agencies and pharmaceutical companies would eliminate the career incentives that currently encourage regulatory officials to maintain industry-friendly attitudes during their government service.

Mandatory Transparency: Pharmaceutical companies should be required to disclose all manufacturing information, including facility locations, supply chain details, quality control procedures, and safety testing data. Trade secret protections should not override patient safety information needs.

Real-Time Monitoring: Regulatory oversight should include real-time monitoring of pharmaceutical manufacturing rather than relying on infrequent inspections that allow facilities to hide problems between regulatory visits.

Enhanced Enforcement Authority

Regulators need enhanced authority and resources to ensure meaningful compliance with safety standards:

Immediate Shutdown Authority: Regulators should have the authority to immediately halt operations at facilities with serious safety problems rather than relying on slow bureaucratic processes that allow contaminated medications to continue reaching patients.

Meaningful Financial Penalties: Financial penalties for safety violations should be large enough to deter dangerous practices rather than treating safety violations as acceptable business costs. Penalties should be based on company revenue rather than fixed amounts that become insignificant for large corporations.

Criminal Prosecution: Corporate executives who knowingly endanger patient safety should face criminal prosecution rather than just civil penalties. Personal accountability for safety failures would create stronger incentives for corporate safety compliance.

Victim Compensation: Pharmaceutical companies should be required to fund victim compensation systems that provide immediate support for patients harmed by contaminated or defective medications rather than forcing victims to pursue lengthy litigation.

The Manufacturing Standards Revolution

Creating genuinely safe pharmaceutical manufacturing requires implementing standards that prioritize patient protection over cost minimization.

Quality-First Manufacturing Requirements

American pharmaceutical manufacturing should adopt quality-first standards that make safety the primary consideration in all manufacturing decisions:

Contamination Prevention: Manufacturing facilities should be required to implement contamination prevention systems that exceed current standards, with mandatory environmental monitoring and real-time contamination detection.

Supply Chain Control: Companies should be required to maintain direct control over their entire supply chains rather than relying on multiple intermediaries that obscure contamination sources and quality problems.

Batch Tracking: Every medication dose should be traceable to its specific manufacturing batch, raw material sources, and quality control testing results, enabling rapid identification and isolation of problems.

Redundant Safety Systems: Manufacturing facilities should be required to implement redundant safety systems that prevent single points of failure from causing widespread contamination or quality problems.

Domestic Manufacturing Incentives

American pharmaceutical policy should include incentives for maintaining domestic manufacturing capacity while ensuring that overseas facilities meet American safety standards:

Strategic Manufacturing Reserves: Critical medications should be required to maintain domestic manufacturing capacity to prevent supply disruptions and ensure access to American-standard manufacturing.

Tax Incentives: Companies that maintain domestic manufacturing with enhanced safety standards should receive tax incentives that offset the additional costs of genuine safety compliance.

Procurement Preferences: Government procurement programs should prioritize medications manufactured under enhanced safety standards rather than simply choosing the lowest-cost options.

Import Standards: Foreign-manufactured medications should be required to meet the same safety standards as domestically produced medications, with equivalent inspection frequency and quality oversight.

The Political Action Framework

Achieving meaningful pharmaceutical safety reform requires sustained political action that overcomes industry resistance and creates genuine accountability for patient safety.

Legislative Priorities

Specific legislative changes are needed to create the regulatory framework for pharmaceutical safety reform:

The Pharmaceutical Safety Act: Comprehensive legislation should establish patient safety as the primary purpose of pharmaceutical regulation, with specific requirements for safety testing, contamination prevention, and patient notification.

The Manufacturing Transparency Act: Legislation requiring complete disclosure of pharmaceutical manufacturing information would enable meaningful oversight and patient decision-making about medication safety.

The Regulatory Independence Act: Legislation eliminating pharmaceutical industry funding of regulatory oversight would create the independence necessary for genuine safety regulation.

The Patient Protection Act: Legislation establishing comprehensive patient rights in pharmaceutical safety would ensure that safety considerations take precedence over industry convenience in regulatory decisions.

Electoral Strategy

Pharmaceutical safety reform requires electing representatives who prioritize patient safety over pharmaceutical industry campaign contributions:

Candidate Evaluation: Voters should evaluate candidates based on their positions on pharmaceutical safety reform and their history of independence from pharmaceutical industry influence.

Issue Priority: Pharmaceutical safety should become a priority issue in political campaigns, with candidates required to take specific positions on reform proposals.

Campaign Finance Reform: Broader campaign finance reforms are needed to reduce pharmaceutical industry influence over elected officials and regulatory appointees.

Grassroots Organization: Patient advocacy organizations need to develop grassroots political power that can compete with pharmaceutical industry lobbying and campaign contributions.

The Economic Transformation Strategy

Creating sustainable pharmaceutical safety requires recognizing that genuine safety is economically beneficial rather than economically burdensome.

The True Cost of Unsafe Medications

Current pharmaceutical economics ignore the massive hidden costs of unsafe medications that are borne by patients and healthcare systems rather than pharmaceutical companies:

Healthcare System Costs: Adverse events from contaminated medications, medication errors, and pharmaceutical-related health problems represent billions in healthcare costs that could be prevented through better manufacturing and safety standards.

Lost Productivity: Pharmaceutical-related health problems cause massive losses in worker productivity and economic output that exceed the costs of implementing better safety systems.

Legal System Costs: The current system's reliance on litigation to address pharmaceutical safety problems creates enormous legal costs that could be eliminated through prevention-focused safety systems.

Innovation Opportunities: Investment in pharmaceutical safety technology and manufacturing excellence could create new industries and economic opportunities while improving patient outcomes.

Market-Based Safety Incentives

Economic incentives can be restructured to reward safety excellence rather than cost-cutting that endangers patients:

Safety-Based Pricing: Insurance companies and government programs should base medication reimbursement on safety records rather than just cost considerations, creating market incentives for safety excellence.

Liability Insurance Requirements: Pharmaceutical companies should be required to maintain liability insurance that reflects the true costs of safety failures, internalizing the costs of dangerous practices.

Quality Certification Programs: Independent quality certification programs could provide market differentiation for companies that exceed minimum safety standards, creating competitive advantages for safety excellence.

Consumer Safety Information: Comprehensive safety information should be readily available to patients and healthcare providers, enabling market forces to reward safer medications through informed consumer choice.

The Technology Solutions

Modern technology provides opportunities for dramatically improving pharmaceutical safety while reducing costs and improving efficiency.

Advanced Manufacturing Technology

New manufacturing technologies can eliminate many contamination sources while improving quality consistency:

Continuous Manufacturing: Advanced manufacturing systems that provide real-time quality monitoring and contamination detection can prevent problems from affecting large numbers of medication doses.

Automated Quality Control: Artificial intelligence and machine learning systems can identify quality problems and contamination patterns that human oversight might miss.

Blockchain Supply Chains: Blockchain technology can provide complete supply chain transparency and traceability that enables rapid identification of contamination sources and quality problems.

Remote Monitoring: Real-time monitoring systems can provide continuous oversight of manufacturing operations rather than relying on periodic inspections that allow problems to persist between regulatory visits.

Patient Safety Technology

Technology solutions can also improve patient safety through better information and monitoring:

Medication Safety Apps: Smartphone applications can provide real-time safety information, recall alerts, and quality monitoring that keeps patients informed about their medication safety.

Electronic Health Record Integration: Safety information should be automatically integrated into electronic health records so that healthcare providers and patients receive immediate alerts about safety problems affecting their medications.

Pharmacogenetic Testing: Widespread availability of genetic testing for medication metabolism could reduce adverse effects by identifying patients who are likely to have problems with specific medications or manufacturing processes.

Artificial Intelligence Monitoring: AI systems could monitor patient reports and healthcare data to identify safety patterns that might indicate contamination or quality problems before they're officially recognized.

The Personal Responsibility Framework

While systemic reform is essential, individuals also have responsibilities for supporting pharmaceutical safety reform and protecting their own health within the current flawed system.

Individual Action Steps

Every patient can contribute to pharmaceutical safety reform while protecting their own health:

Political Engagement: Contact elected representatives about pharmaceutical safety concerns and support candidates who prioritize patient safety over pharmaceutical industry interests.

Healthcare Provider Education: Educate healthcare providers about pharmaceutical safety concerns and demand consideration of safety factors in treatment decisions.

Consumer Choice: Use your purchasing power to support companies with better safety records and avoid products from manufacturers with inferior quality histories.

Information Sharing: Share your knowledge about pharmaceutical safety with family, friends, and community members to build broader awareness and support for reform.

Advocacy Support: Support patient advocacy organizations that prioritize genuine safety reform over pharmaceutical industry funding and influence.

Community Organization

Building community support for pharmaceutical safety reform requires organized efforts that create political pressure for change:

Local Advocacy Groups: Organize local groups focused on pharmaceutical safety and healthcare reform that can influence local political representatives and healthcare institutions.

Healthcare Institution Pressure: Work with local hospitals, clinics, and healthcare systems to implement higher safety standards and more comprehensive patient protection policies.

Media Engagement: Work with local media to increase coverage of pharmaceutical safety issues and create public pressure for reform.

Educational Programs: Develop community education programs that help other patients understand pharmaceutical safety issues and protect themselves from current system failures.

The Vision for Pharmaceutical Excellence

The ultimate goal of pharmaceutical safety reform should be creating a system that serves patients rather than exploiting them, that prioritizes health outcomes over financial returns, and that treats medication safety as a fundamental right rather than a luxury for those who can afford it.

The Patient-Centered System

A reformed pharmaceutical system would prioritize patient welfare in every aspect of medication development, manufacturing, and distribution:

Transparent Manufacturing: Patients would have complete information about how their medications are manufactured, where they come from, and what safety testing has been conducted.

Genuine Choice: Patients would have access to multiple safe alternatives for their medical conditions rather than being forced to accept whatever options insurance companies and healthcare systems find most profitable.

Comprehensive Safety: Every medication would be tested for safety as a complete formulation rather than just as individual active ingredients, with ongoing monitoring for long-term effects and contamination risks.

Rapid Response: Safety problems would be identified and addressed immediately rather than being allowed to persist while bureaucratic processes protect industry interests over patient safety.

The Innovation Imperative

A safety-focused pharmaceutical system would drive innovation in manufacturing technology, quality control, and patient protection rather than stifling innovation through excessive regulation:

Safety Technology Development: Investment in safety technology and quality control systems would create new industries and economic opportunities while improving patient outcomes.

Precision Medicine: Better understanding of individual patient responses to medications would enable more targeted and safer treatments while reducing adverse effects from inappropriate medication choices.

Prevention Focus: Emphasis on preventing health problems rather than just treating them would reduce overall medication needs while improving population health outcomes.

Global Leadership: American leadership in pharmaceutical safety could create export opportunities for safety technology and establish American companies as global leaders in pharmaceutical excellence.

The Urgency of Action

The pharmaceutical safety crisis is not a future threat—it's a present reality that affects millions of Americans every day. Every day we delay implementing meaningful reforms, more patients are exposed to preventable risks from contaminated medications, dangerous chemical additives, and systemic quality failures.

The cost of inaction far exceeds the cost of reform. The current system's hidden costs—in healthcare expenses, lost productivity, damaged health, and eroded public trust—represent a massive economic burden that could be eliminated through prevention-focused safety reforms.

More importantly, the human cost of continued inaction is unacceptable. Every patient who suffers adverse effects from contaminated medications, every family that struggles with medication-related health problems, and every individual who loses faith in the healthcare system represents a moral failure that demands immediate action.

The pharmaceutical industry will not reform itself. Companies that prioritize profits over patient safety will continue doing so until they're forced to change through regulatory requirements, market pressure, and political action. Creating that pressure requires sustained effort from patients, healthcare providers, advocacy organizations, and political leaders who prioritize public health over industry convenience.

The Choice Before Us

We face a fundamental choice about the kind of healthcare system we want in America. We can continue accepting a pharmaceutical system that treats patient safety as an obstacle to profitability, or we can demand a system that treats patient welfare as its primary purpose.

The choice isn't between medication access and medication safety—other countries have proven that we can have both. The choice is between accepting a system designed to enrich pharmaceutical companies at patients' expense, or demanding a system designed to serve patients while maintaining reasonable industry profitability.

The path forward requires acknowledging that pharmaceutical safety is a political issue that demands political solutions. Individual patients can protect themselves through vigilance and advocacy, but systemic change requires collective action that forces fundamental reforms in how medications are manufactured, regulated, and distributed.

The pharmaceutical industry has spent decades building a system that serves their interests while exploiting patients. Dismantling that system and replacing it with genuine patient protection will require sustained effort from everyone who believes that healthcare should heal rather than harm.

The journey I began following my surgeries and medication discoveries has convinced me that change is possible, but only if we're willing to demand it. The evidence of systematic pharmaceutical failures is overwhelming, the solutions are available, and the moral imperative for action is clear.

The question isn't whether we can build a better system—it's whether we will. The answer depends on whether patients, healthcare providers, and political leaders are willing to prioritize human health over pharmaceutical industry profits. Your voice, your vote, and your advocacy can help determine that answer.

The path forward begins with each of us refusing to accept a system that treats our health as less important than corporate profits. It continues with demanding transparency, accountability, and genuine safety from every aspect of the pharmaceutical system. And it culminates in building a healthcare system that serves patients rather than exploiting them.

That transformation won't happen automatically, and it won't happen quickly. But it can happen, and it must happen, because our health and our lives depend on it. The pharmaceutical industry has had decades to prove they can regulate themselves responsibly. They've failed that test repeatedly and catastrophically.

Now it's time for the rest of us to take back control of our healthcare and demand the safe, effective, transparent pharmaceutical system we deserve. The path forward is clear—the only question is whether we have the courage to walk it.

Conclusion: Your Journey Toward Pharmaceutical Safety

Thank you for joining me on this investigative journey into the hidden world of pharmaceutical contamination and chemical dangers. When I began researching the soy and dairy I discovered in my medications after 18 surgeries, I never imagined it would lead to uncovering a systematic crisis affecting millions of Americans who trust their medications to heal rather than harm.

The evidence presented in this book reveals uncomfortable truths about an industry that has prioritized profits over patient safety for far too long. From contaminated manufacturing facilities in China and India to regulatory agencies captured by the companies they're supposed to oversee, from hidden allergens in everyday medications to recall systems designed to protect companies rather than patients—the scope of the pharmaceutical safety crisis is both shocking and undeniable.

But this book isn't just about exposing problems—it's about empowering you to protect yourself and your family while advocating for the systemic changes we desperately need. The strategies outlined in Chapters 12 and 13 represent practical steps that any patient can implement immediately to reduce their exposure to pharmaceutical dangers. The reform framework presented in Chapter 14 provides a roadmap for the political and regulatory changes necessary to create a pharmaceutical system that truly serves patients rather than exploiting them.

The Power of Informed Patients

Your safety ultimately depends on your own knowledge, vigilance, and advocacy. The pharmaceutical industry and regulatory agencies have repeatedly demonstrated that they cannot be trusted to prioritize patient welfare over corporate profits. By becoming an informed, empowered patient who asks the right questions, demands transparency, and makes thoughtful decisions about medication choices, you can protect yourself while contributing to broader efforts for systemic reform.

Remember that every time you research a medication's manufacturer, ask your pharmacist about contamination risks, or demand safer alternatives from your healthcare provider, you're not just protecting your own health—you're helping to build market pressure for pharmaceutical companies to prioritize safety over convenience.

The Urgency of Collective Action

Individual protection is essential, but systemic change requires collective action. The pharmaceutical industry's influence over regulatory agencies, academic research, and political processes can only be overcome through sustained pressure from informed patients, healthcare providers, and political leaders who prioritize public health over industry convenience.

Support patient advocacy organizations that genuinely prioritize safety over pharmaceutical industry funding. Contact your elected representatives about pharmaceutical safety concerns. Share this information with family, friends, and community members to build broader awareness of these critical issues. Use your purchasing power and political voice to demand the pharmaceutical system we deserve—one that treats patient safety as a fundamental right rather than a luxury for those who can afford it.

A Personal Note

This investigation has fundamentally changed how I approach healthcare decisions, and I hope it changes how you approach them as well. The comfortable assumption that someone else is protecting our medication safety has been replaced by the knowledge that we must protect ourselves through vigilance, advocacy, and informed decision-making.

The journey isn't always easy, but the alternative—continuing to accept a system that treats our health as less important than corporate profits—is unacceptable. We deserve better, our families deserve better, and future generations deserve a pharmaceutical system that genuinely serves patients rather than exploiting them.

Thank you for taking the time to learn about these critical issues. Your awareness and advocacy can help build the momentum necessary for meaningful change. Together, we can demand and create a pharmaceutical system worthy of our trust.

Other Books in Kevin's Health Investigation Series

If you found "Unsafe at Any Dose" eye-opening, you'll want to explore the other shocking truths about the hidden dangers in our environment and food supply. Kevin's investigative series exposes the chemical contamination affecting every aspect of our daily lives:

"Microplastics: The Invisible Invasion"

The Hidden Plastic Contamination in Our Bodies and Environment

Discover the shocking truth about how microplastics from packaging, clothing, and industrial processes are contaminating our food, water, and even the air we breathe. Learn how these invisible particles are accumulating in human tissues and what you can do to minimize your exposure.

"Bad Air: The Chemical Assault on Our Lungs"

What the Air Quality Index Doesn't Tell You

Uncover the hidden air pollutants that government monitoring ignores—from volatile organic compounds in household products to industrial chemicals that drift for miles. This investigation reveals how indoor air is often more toxic than outdoor air and provides practical strategies for protecting your family.

"Chemicals in Our Food: The Pesticide and Additive Crisis"

What Food Labels Don't Reveal About What You're Really Eating

Expose the chemical reality of modern food production, from pesticide residues that persist despite washing to artificial additives that serve corporate profits rather than nutritional needs. Learn how to navigate the toxic food landscape and make safer choices for your family.

The Complete Series Available:

Online retailers: Amazon, Barnes & Noble, Apple Books

Physical bookstores: Available worldwide through major book retailers

Libraries: Request these titles at your local library

International: Available in multiple countries and formats

Each book in the series follows the same investigative approach used in "Unsafe at Any Dose"—combining personal experience with rigorous research to expose hidden dangers while providing practical protection strategies. Together, these books provide a comprehensive guide to navigating the chemical hazards of modern life.

Stay Connected

For updates on pharmaceutical safety issues and information about new investigations, visit [author website information would go here]. Join the community of informed consumers who are demanding transparency and safety in the products that affect our health.

Your health is too important to leave to others. Take control, stay informed, and demand better.

All books in Kevin's Health Investigation Series are available at major book retailers worldwide. Check your local bookstore or preferred online retailer for availability and current pricing.

The pharmaceutical industry has spent decades building a system that serves their interests while exploiting patients. Dismantling that system and replacing it with genuine patient protection will require sustained effort from everyone who believes that healthcare should heal rather than harm.

The evidence is overwhelming, the solutions are available, and the moral imperative for action is clear. The question isn't whether we can build a better system—it's whether we will. The answer depends on whether patients, healthcare providers, and political leaders are willing to prioritize human health over pharmaceutical industry profits.

Your voice, your vote, and your advocacy can help determine that answer. The path forward begins with each of us refusing to accept a system that treats our health as less important than corporate profits. The time for action is now.

Sources and Further Reading

The information in this book is based on publicly available government documents, peer-reviewed research, regulatory databases, and official industry communications. All sources listed below can be independently verified online. Readers are encouraged to examine these sources directly and conduct their own research into pharmaceutical safety issues.

Government and Regulatory Sources

U.S. Food and Drug Administration (FDA)

FDA Drug Recalls Database: https://www.fda.gov/drugs/drug-recalls

FDA Warning Letters Database: https://www.fda.gov/inspections-compliance-enforcement-and-criminal-investigations/compliance-actions-and-activities/warning-letters

FDA Inspection Reports: https://www.fda.gov/about-fda/reports/fda-reports

FDA Adverse Event Reporting System (FAERS): https://www.fda.gov/drugs/questions-and-answers-fdas-adverse-event-reporting-system-faers/fda-adverse-event-reporting-system-faers-public-dashboard

FDA Generic Drug Program: https://www.fda.gov/drugs/abbreviated-new-drug-application-anda/generic-drugs-questions-answers

FDA Generally Recognized as Safe (GRAS) Database: https://www.fda.gov/food/food-additives-petitions/generally-recognized-safe-gras

Centers for Disease Control and Prevention (CDC)

Medication Safety Program: https://www.cdc.gov/medicationsafety/

Adverse Drug Events: https://www.cdc.gov/medicationsafety/adverse_drug_events.html

Government Accountability Office (GAO)

Drug Safety Reports: https://www.gao.gov/products/gao-09-704

FDA Oversight Reports: https://www.gao.gov/key_issues/food_and_drug_safety/issue_summary

Office of Inspector General - Department of Health and Human Services

FDA Inspection Reports: https://oig.hhs.gov/reports-and-publications/workplan/summary/wp-summary-0000352.asp

International Regulatory Sources

European Medicines Agency (EMA)

Safety Communications: https://www.ema.europa.eu/en/human-regulatory/post-marketing/pharmacovigilance

Good Manufacturing Practice Guidelines: https://www.ema.europa.eu/en/human-regulatory/research-development/compliance/good-manufacturing-practice

Health Canada

Drug Product Database: https://www.canada.ca/en/health-canada/services/drugs-health-products/drug-products/drug-product-database.html

Recalls and Safety Alerts: https://www.canada.ca/en/health-canada/services/drugs-health-products/medeffect-canada/health-product-infowatch.html

World Health Organization (WHO)

Pharmaceutical Quality Assurance: https://www.who.int/teams/health-products-policy-and-standards/standards-and-specifications/norms-and-standards-for-pharmaceuticals

Essential Medicines and Health Products: https://www.who.int/teams/essential-medicines-and-health-products

Peer-Reviewed Research and Academic Sources

PubMed - National Library of Medicine

Database Access: https://pubmed.ncbi.nlm.nih.gov/

Search Terms: "pharmaceutical contamination," "drug safety," "generic drug quality," "NDMA contamination," "pharmaceutical excipients"

Research Topics to Search (Available on PubMed)

Search terms: "NDMA contamination pharmaceutical," "valsartan recall," "nitrosamine drugs"

Search terms: "generic drug quality," "bioequivalence studies," "pharmaceutical manufacturing"

Search terms: "pharmaceutical excipients safety," "inactive ingredients," "drug contamination"

Search terms: "FDA drug recalls," "pharmaceutical quality control," "generic vs brand name"

Cochrane Reviews

Database Access: https://www.cochranelibrary.com/

Reviews on Drug Safety and Quality

Industry and Manufacturing Information

Pharmaceutical Research and Manufacturers of America (PhRMA)

Industry Statistics: https://www.phrma.org/

Manufacturing Guidelines: Available through member company reports

Generic Pharmaceutical Association (Now AAM)

Generic Drug Facts: https://accessiblemeds.org/

Manufacturing Information: Industry white papers and reports

International Council for Harmonisation (ICH)

Quality Guidelines: https://www.ich.org/products/guidelines/quality/article/quality-guidelines.html

Good Manufacturing Practice Guidelines

News and Investigative Reporting

Major News Organizations with Health Coverage

Reuters Health News: Available in Reuters online archives

Associated Press Medical Coverage: Search AP archives for pharmaceutical topics

ProPublica Health Investigations: https://www.propublica.org/ (search health/pharmaceutical topics)

Kaiser Health News: https://khn.org/ - Independent health journalism

Trade Publications

Pharmaceutical Technology Magazine: https://www.pharmtech.com/

FDA News: https://www.fdanews.com/

Pink Sheet (Pharma Intelligence): Industry regulatory news

Legal and Litigation Sources

Court Documents and Legal Filings

PACER Database: https://pacer.uscourts.gov/ - Federal court records

SEC Filing Database: https://www.sec.gov/edgar - Corporate disclosure documents

Class Action Lawsuits: Available through legal databases and court records

Department of Justice

Criminal and Civil Cases: https://www.justice.gov/opa/pr - Press releases on pharmaceutical prosecutions

Settlement Agreements: Available through DOJ archives

Patient Safety and Advocacy Organizations

Institute for Safe Medication Practices (ISMP)

Safety Alerts: https://www.ismp.org/

Medication Error Reports: https://www.ismp.org/recommendations

Patient Safety Organizations

The Leapfrog Group: https://www.leapfroggroup.org/

National Patient Safety Foundation: Resources and reports

Consumer Advocacy

Public Citizen Health Research Group: https://www.citizen.org/our-work/health-and-safety/

Consumer Reports Drug Safety: https://www.consumerreports.org/health/

Pharmaceutical Industry Databases

FDA Orange Book

Approved Drug Products: https://www.fda.gov/drugs/drug-approvals-and-databases/approved-drug-products-therapeutic-equivalence-evaluations-orange-book

National Drug Code Directory

Drug Identification: https://www.fda.gov/drugs/drug-approvals-and-databases/national-drug-code-directory

Drug Manufacturer Information

FDA Establishment Registration: https://www.fda.gov/drugs/registration-and-listing-guidance-industry/establishment-registration-and-drug-listing-guidance-industry

Scientific and Technical Resources

American Chemical Society

Chemical Safety Information: https://www.acs.org/

Pharmaceutical Chemistry Research

International Pharmaceutical Federation (FIP)

Global Pharmacy Reports: https://www.fip.org/

Quality Assurance Guidelines

United States Pharmacopeia (USP)

Drug Standards: https://www.usp.org/

Quality Control Guidelines: https://www.usp.org/quality-control

Contamination-Specific Resources

NDMA and Nitrosamine Contamination

FDA Guidance Documents: https://www.fda.gov/drugs/drug-safety-and-availability/updates-and-press-announcements-angiotensin-ii-receptor-blocker-arb-recalls-valsartan-losartan

European Assessment Reports: Available through EMA website

Scientific Literature: Available through PubMed using search terms "NDMA pharmaceutical contamination"

Heavy Metal Contamination

EPA Guidelines: https://www.epa.gov/metals-food-and-drugs

FDA Heavy Metal Testing: Available through FDA guidance documents

Manufacturing and Supply Chain Information

FDA Facility Inspection Reports

Domestic Facilities: Available through FDA databases

Foreign Facility Reports: https://www.fda.gov/about-fda/reports/fda-reports

Supply Chain Transparency

Corporate Annual Reports: Available through SEC EDGAR database

Sustainability Reports: Available on pharmaceutical company websites

Healthcare Economics and Policy

Centers for Medicare & Medicaid Services (CMS)

Drug Spending Data: https://www.cms.gov/Research-Statistics-Data-and-Systems/Statistics-Trends-and-Reports/Information-on-Prescription-Drugs

Medicare Part D Data: https://www.cms.gov/Research-Statistics-Data-and-Systems/Statistics-Trends-and-Reports/Medicare-Provider-Charge-Data/Part-D-Prescriber

Congressional Research Service

Pharmaceutical Policy Reports: Available through government document repositories

Drug Safety Oversight Reports

How to Use These Sources

Research Strategies

Start with government databases for official information on recalls, inspections, and safety alerts

Cross-reference multiple sources to verify information and identify patterns

Use PubMed for peer-reviewed scientific research on specific safety topics

Check international sources to compare safety standards and practices

Review court documents for detailed information about industry practices revealed through litigation

Staying Current

Set up Google Alerts for pharmaceutical safety topics

Subscribe to FDA safety alerts and recall notifications

Monitor patient advocacy websites for emerging safety concerns

Follow investigative journalists who cover pharmaceutical industry issues

Check international regulatory websites for early warnings about safety problems

Verification Guidelines

Prefer primary sources over secondary reporting when possible

Check publication dates to ensure information is current

Verify author credentials and potential conflicts of interest

Cross-reference claims across multiple independent sources

Distinguish between correlation and causation in research reports

Important Disclaimers

Source Limitations

Government databases may not include all safety information due to reporting gaps

Industry sources may present information in ways that minimize apparent risks

Academic research may be limited by funding sources and publication bias

News reporting may oversimplify complex technical issues

Legal documents represent allegations that may not have been proven in court

Research Considerations

Publication bias may mean negative results are underreported

Funding sources can influence research design and interpretation

Regulatory capture may affect the completeness of government oversight information

Industry influence on academic research and professional organizations

Time delays between problem identification and public disclosure

Using Information Responsibly

Consult healthcare providers before making medication decisions based on safety concerns

Consider individual risk factors when evaluating general safety information

Distinguish between theoretical risks and documented harms

Understand that correlation does not prove causation

Recognize that medication benefits may outweigh identified risks

Recommended Further Reading

Books on Healthcare and Pharmaceutical Issues

Available through libraries and bookstores - readers should verify current availability

Topics to research: pharmaceutical industry practices, drug safety, healthcare policy

Academic and trade books on pharmaceutical manufacturing and regulation

Academic Journals

Journal of Pharmaceutical Sciences

Pharmaceutical Research

Drug Safety

Clinical Pharmacology & Therapeutics

The Lancet

New England Journal of Medicine

Professional Organizations

American Society of Health-System Pharmacists (ASHP): https://www.ashp.org/

International Society for Pharmaceutical Engineering (ISPE): https://ispe.org/

Parenteral Drug Association (PDA): https://www.pda.org/

Note to Readers: This source list provides starting points for independent research into pharmaceutical safety issues. The pharmaceutical industry and regulatory landscape change rapidly, so readers should always seek the most current information available. When making healthcare decisions, consult with qualified healthcare providers who can help interpret safety information in the context of individual medical needs and circumstances.

The author encourages readers to become informed advocates for their own health while recognizing that medication decisions involve complex risk-benefit calculations that should be made in consultation with healthcare professionals who understand individual medical circumstances.

Sources and Further Reading

The information in this book is based on publicly available government documents, peer-reviewed research, regulatory databases, and official industry communications. All sources listed below can be independently verified online. Readers are encouraged to examine these sources directly and conduct their own research into pharmaceutical safety issues.

Government and Regulatory Sources

U.S. Food and Drug Administration (FDA)

FDA Drug Recalls Database: https://www.fda.gov/drugs/drug-recalls

FDA Warning Letters Database: https://www.fda.gov/inspections-compliance-enforcement-and-criminal-investigations/compliance-actions-and-activities/warning-letters

FDA Inspection Reports: https://www.fda.gov/about-fda/reports/fda-reports

FDA Adverse Event Reporting System (FAERS): https://www.fda.gov/drugs/questions-and-answers-fdas-adverse-event-reporting-system-faers/fda-adverse-event-reporting-system-faers-public-dashboard

FDA Generic Drug Program:
https://www.fda.gov/drugs/abbreviated-new-drug-application-anda/generic-drugs-questions-answers

FDA Generally Recognized as Safe (GRAS) Database:
https://www.fda.gov/food/food-additives-petitions/generally-recognized-safe-gras

Centers for Disease Control and Prevention (CDC)

Medication Safety Program:
https://www.cdc.gov/medicationsafety/

Adverse Drug Events:
https://www.cdc.gov/medicationsafety/adverse_drug_events.html

Government Accountability Office (GAO)

Drug Safety Reports: https://www.gao.gov/products/gao-09-704

FDA Oversight Reports:
https://www.gao.gov/key_issues/food_and_drug_safety/issue_summary

Office of Inspector General - Department of Health and Human Services

FDA Inspection Reports: https://oig.hhs.gov/reports-and-publications/workplan/summary/wp-summary-0000352.asp

International Regulatory Sources

European Medicines Agency (EMA)

Safety Communications: https://www.ema.europa.eu/en/human-regulatory/post-marketing/pharmacovigilance

Good Manufacturing Practice Guidelines: https://www.ema.europa.eu/en/human-regulatory/research-development/compliance/good-manufacturing-practice

Health Canada

Drug Product Database: https://www.canada.ca/en/health-canada/services/drugs-health-products/drug-products/drug-product-database.html

Recalls and Safety Alerts: https://www.canada.ca/en/health-canada/services/drugs-health-products/medeffect-canada/health-product-infowatch.html

World Health Organization (WHO)

Pharmaceutical Quality Assurance: https://www.who.int/teams/health-products-policy-and-standards/standards-and-specifications/norms-and-standards-for-pharmaceuticals

Essential Medicines and Health Products: https://www.who.int/teams/essential-medicines-and-health-products

Peer-Reviewed Research and Academic Sources

PubMed - National Library of Medicine

Database Access: https://pubmed.ncbi.nlm.nih.gov/

Search Terms: "pharmaceutical contamination," "drug safety," "generic drug quality," "NDMA contamination," "pharmaceutical excipients"

Research Topics to Search (Available on PubMed)

Search terms: "NDMA contamination pharmaceutical," "valsartan recall," "nitrosamine drugs"

Search terms: "generic drug quality," "bioequivalence studies," "pharmaceutical manufacturing"

Search terms: "pharmaceutical excipients safety," "inactive ingredients," "drug contamination"

Search terms: "FDA drug recalls," "pharmaceutical quality control," "generic vs brand name"

Cochrane Reviews

Database Access: https://www.cochranelibrary.com/

Reviews on Drug Safety and Quality

Industry and Manufacturing Information

Pharmaceutical Research and Manufacturers of America (PhRMA)

Industry Statistics: https://www.phrma.org/

Manufacturing Guidelines: Available through member company reports

Generic Pharmaceutical Association (Now AAM)

Generic Drug Facts: https://accessiblemeds.org/

Manufacturing Information: Industry white papers and reports

International Council for Harmonisation (ICH)

Quality Guidelines: https://www.ich.org/products/guidelines/quality/article/quality-guidelines.html

Good Manufacturing Practice Guidelines

News and Investigative Reporting

Major News Organizations with Health Coverage

Reuters Health News: Available in Reuters online archives

Associated Press Medical Coverage: Search AP archives for pharmaceutical topics

ProPublica Health Investigations: https://www.propublica.org/ (search health/pharmaceutical topics)

Kaiser Health News: https://khn.org/ - Independent health journalism

Trade Publications

Pharmaceutical Technology Magazine: https://www.pharmtech.com/

FDA News: https://www.fdanews.com/

Pink Sheet (Pharma Intelligence): Industry regulatory news

Legal and Litigation Sources

Court Documents and Legal Filings

PACER Database: https://pacer.uscourts.gov/ - Federal court records

SEC Filing Database: https://www.sec.gov/edgar - Corporate disclosure documents

Class Action Lawsuits: Available through legal databases and court records

Department of Justice

Criminal and Civil Cases: https://www.justice.gov/opa/pr - Press releases on pharmaceutical prosecutions

Settlement Agreements: Available through DOJ archives

Patient Safety and Advocacy Organizations

Institute for Safe Medication Practices (ISMP)

Safety Alerts: https://www.ismp.org/

Medication Error Reports: https://www.ismp.org/recommendations

Patient Safety Organizations

The Leapfrog Group: https://www.leapfroggroup.org/

National Patient Safety Foundation: Resources and reports

Consumer Advocacy

Public Citizen Health Research Group: https://www.citizen.org/our-work/health-and-safety/

Consumer Reports Drug Safety: https://www.consumerreports.org/health/

Pharmaceutical Industry Databases

FDA Orange Book

Approved Drug Products: https://www.fda.gov/drugs/drug-approvals-and-databases/approved-drug-products-therapeutic-equivalence-evaluations-orange-book

National Drug Code Directory

Drug Identification: https://www.fda.gov/drugs/drug-approvals-and-databases/national-drug-code-directory

Drug Manufacturer Information

FDA Establishment Registration: https://www.fda.gov/drugs/registration-and-listing-guidance-industry/establishment-registration-and-drug-listing-guidance-industry

Scientific and Technical Resources

American Chemical Society

Chemical Safety Information: https://www.acs.org/

Pharmaceutical Chemistry Research

International Pharmaceutical Federation (FIP)

Global Pharmacy Reports: https://www.fip.org/

Quality Assurance Guidelines

United States Pharmacopeia (USP)

Drug Standards: https://www.usp.org/

Quality Control Guidelines: https://www.usp.org/quality-control

Contamination-Specific Resources

NDMA and Nitrosamine Contamination

FDA Guidance Documents: https://www.fda.gov/drugs/drug-safety-and-availability/updates-and-press-announcements-angiotensin-ii-receptor-blocker-arb-recalls-valsartan-losartan

European Assessment Reports: Available through EMA website

Scientific Literature: Available through PubMed using search terms "NDMA pharmaceutical contamination"

Heavy Metal Contamination

EPA Guidelines: https://www.epa.gov/metals-food-and-drugs

FDA Heavy Metal Testing: Available through FDA guidance documents

Manufacturing and Supply Chain Information

FDA Facility Inspection Reports

Domestic Facilities: Available through FDA databases

Foreign Facility Reports: https://www.fda.gov/about-fda/reports/fda-reports

Supply Chain Transparency

Corporate Annual Reports: Available through SEC EDGAR database

Sustainability Reports: Available on pharmaceutical company websites

Healthcare Economics and Policy

Centers for Medicare & Medicaid Services (CMS)

Drug Spending Data: https://www.cms.gov/Research-Statistics-Data-and-Systems/Statistics-Trends-and-Reports/Information-on-Prescription-Drugs

Medicare Part D Data: https://www.cms.gov/Research-Statistics-Data-and-Systems/Statistics-Trends-and-Reports/Medicare-Provider-Charge-Data/Part-D-Prescriber

Congressional Research Service

Pharmaceutical Policy Reports: Available through government document repositories

Drug Safety Oversight Reports

How to Use These Sources

Research Strategies

Start with government databases for official information on recalls, inspections, and safety alerts

Cross-reference multiple sources to verify information and identify patterns

Use PubMed for peer-reviewed scientific research on specific safety topics

Check international sources to compare safety standards and practices

Review court documents for detailed information about industry practices revealed through litigation

Staying Current

Set up Google Alerts for pharmaceutical safety topics

Subscribe to FDA safety alerts and recall notifications

Monitor patient advocacy websites for emerging safety concerns

Follow investigative journalists who cover pharmaceutical industry issues

Check international regulatory websites for early warnings about safety problems

Verification Guidelines

Prefer primary sources over secondary reporting when possible

Check publication dates to ensure information is current

Verify author credentials and potential conflicts of interest

Cross-reference claims across multiple independent sources

Distinguish between correlation and causation in research reports

Important Disclaimers

Source Limitations

Government databases may not include all safety information due to reporting gaps

Industry sources may present information in ways that minimize apparent risks

Academic research may be limited by funding sources and publication bias

News reporting may oversimplify complex technical issues

Legal documents represent allegations that may not have been proven in court

Research Considerations

Publication bias may mean negative results are underreported

Funding sources can influence research design and interpretation

Regulatory capture may affect the completeness of government oversight information

Industry influence on academic research and professional organizations

Time delays between problem identification and public disclosure

Using Information Responsibly

Consult healthcare providers before making medication decisions based on safety concerns

Consider individual risk factors when evaluating general safety information

Distinguish between theoretical risks and documented harms

Understand that correlation does not prove causation

Recognize that medication benefits may outweigh identified risks

Recommended Further Reading

Books on Healthcare and Pharmaceutical Issues

Available through libraries and bookstores - readers should verify current availability

Topics to research: pharmaceutical industry practices, drug safety, healthcare policy

Academic and trade books on pharmaceutical manufacturing and regulation

Academic Journals

Journal of Pharmaceutical Sciences

Pharmaceutical Research

Drug Safety

Clinical Pharmacology & Therapeutics

The Lancet

New England Journal of Medicine

Professional Organizations

American Society of Health-System Pharmacists (ASHP): https://www.ashp.org/

International Society for Pharmaceutical Engineering (ISPE): https://ispe.org/

Parenteral Drug Association (PDA): https://www.pda.org/

www.ingramcontent.com/pod-product-compliance
Lightning Source LLC
LaVergne TN
LVHW011929070526
838202LV00054B/4549